Loyal Dexter Rogers, Ida Wright Rogers

Rogers' Homeopathic Guide

Loyal Dexter Rogers, Ida Wright Rogers

Rogers' Homeopathic Guide

ISBN/EAN: 9783337372651

Printed in Europe, USA, Canada, Australia, Japan

Cover: Foto ©Lupo / pixelio.de

More available books at **www.hansebooks.com**

ROGERS'
HOMEOPATHIC GUIDE,

A popular treatise, containing a brief description of all diseases, with practical hints for their prevention and cure. Designed for the guidance of intelligent laymen; also, for the ready reference of students and practitioners.

—— BY ——

L. D. ROGERS, A. M., M. D.,

Editor of "The People's Health Journal," Ex-President of the National Medical College, Professor of Surgery in the same, Founder of the Chicago Baptist Hospital, Surgeon to Cook County Hospital, Chicago; author of "Surgical Cleanliness, author of "Homeopathy Explained," Member of the American Institute of Homeopathy, Member of the Illinois Homeopathic Association, a [of] the Homeopathic Society of Chicago;

—— AND ——

IDA WRIGHT ROGERS, M. D.

THIRD EDITION.

...CHICAGO...
THE PEOPLE'S HEALTH JOURNAL COMPANY,
1896.

TO OUR MOTHER,

ELIZABETH JANE PECK ROGERS,

THIS VOLUME

IS AFFECTIONATELY DEDICATED,

ON

HER SIXTY-SECOND BIRTHDAY,

May, 26, 1893.

INTRODUCTION.

TO THE PUBLIC:

Enthusiastic as a student, brilliant, yet thorough, in scholarship, a constant toiler in his profession, successful in organizing results, and devoted to the physical, mental and moral development of society, Dr. L. D. Rogers has won high rank in the city of the Northwest. With a genius remarkable for his profession, a varied talent that touches many lines, an experience already large in hospital and home, a keen and discriminating judgment, he brings the result of all into this *work*.

The author, working side by side with the estimable and accomplished wife, in the reciprocal relation of equal power, proficiency and success, holding with her the golden key of humanity's highest development as regards *man* and *woman*, he has, and holds, the position from which such a work should eminate.

These twain, I imagine, have given to the profession, to the home and the laity in general, in this volume, an exponent of the things needed by all, and to this venture, all who know them, will wish the largest success.

HENRY A. DELANO,

Pres. Board of Directors of the Chicago Baptist Hospital.

Evanston, Ill.

Preface to The Third Edition

THE second edition of this work was exhausted six months ago. Professional duties have occupied our time so completely that we have been unable to prepare the third edition until now. We are pleased to note that this edition is substantially the same as the second, which was so complete that it could not be improved without writing a new and greatly enlarged volume.

The chapter, "Homeopathy Explained," has been revised and published as a separate volume. The chapter on Surgery has been expanded and will appear shortly, also as a separate book, with the title "Surgical Cleanliness."

While there has been continual progress in all departments of medicine and surgery, the advances have not been sufficiently great to materially change the teachings of this book as originally written.

NOVEMBER 15, 1895.   THE AUTHORS.

Preface to the Second Edition.

LESS than ten months ago the first edition of this work was printed. Its rapid sale during a period of the greatest financial depression ever known in this country, and during a period equally remarkable for good health everywhere, is a source of no little gratification. The great popularity of the work has made the authors desirous of improving it. An appendix, therefore, has been added, consisting of two chapters — one, entitled "Homeopathy Explained," and the other, "Supposed Incurables." These should be read first of all. The more important typographical errors in the first edition have been corrected in this one and the table of "errata" omitted. It will be of interest to the agent and to the purchasers to note that at the end of the book a "Coupon" is bound with each copy.

CHICAGO, April 1, 1894.   THE AUTHORS.

PREFACE.

The highest mission of the physician is to prevent disease. In no other way can so much be accomplished toward prevention as by widely disseminating a knowledge of the cause, nature and proper treatment of the various diseases that afflict humanity. A knowledge of the cause of a disease is half the cure and often all the prevention necessary. A knowlege of its nature leads to a correct appreciation of the physician's skill and services. A knowledge of the proper treatment prevents the innocent from being imposed upon by ignorance and quackery. While the practitioner may gain some practical hints from it, this volume is intended as a **guide** to the intelligent layman. It is not intended to make a physician out of him, but to give that general knowledge which every intelligent person should possess.

The progress in medicine and surgery has been so great during the past decade that a medical book, if but three years old, is greatly behind the times and comparatively worthless. The reader may rest assured that this work is up to date and much more recent than any similar work. It also contains much heretofore not attempted in other works. The attention of the reader is called to the sections on Affections of the Mind, Diseases of the Skin, Principles of

INDEX OF CONTENTS.

PAGES.

General Remarks .... 3—10

PART I.

Section I, Constitutional Diseases, Infectious............. 11—115
Section II, Constitutional Diseases, Non-Infectious......... 116—130
Section III, Diseases of the Digestive System............. 131—149
Section IV, Diseases of the Respiratory System........... 150—174
Section V, Diseases of the Circulatory System............ 175—184
Section VII, Diseases of the Kidneys..................... 185—203
Section VIII, Diseases of the Sexual System.............. 204—219
Section IX, Diseases of the Nervous system.............. 220—235
Section X, Unclassified Affections....................... 236—243
Section XI, Affections of the Mind...................... 244—250
Section XII, Diseases of the Skin....................... 251—265
Section XIII, Diseases of the Eye and Ear............... 266—278
Section XIV, The Principles of Surgery.................. 279—292
Section XV, Mother and Child........................... 293—302
Section XVI, Dietetics................................. 303—317

PART II.

Materia Medica....................................... 318—339
Index of Subjects..................................... 340—344
Errata... 351

General Remarks.

What is Health?

It is that condition of the physical and mental machinery in which all the parts work easily and harmoniously, each performing its duty without friction or inconvenience. Most persons know when a piece of machinery is out of order, and they also know the importance of repairing it as soon as possible. If the repair is not made promptly irreparable damage is likely to follow prolonged derangement. But few persons, however, recognize the earliest deviations from health. A person may be far from well and yet unaware of the fact. Every person who desires good health should become familiar with the evidences of good health. Any intelligent person can soon learn them.

Evidences of Good Health. A person in good health is cheerful and good natured, their eyes are bright and sparkling, the lips are red and the complexion clear. The hair is soft, oily and glossy. The skin is smooth and velvety, with a pinkish tint; the sleep is sound, dreamless and refreshing. The appetite is good and no distress of any kind follows eating; no great thirst; no disagreeable taste in the mouth; the tongue is clean and the breath sweet; no belching, no bloating and no flatulency. The bowels move once a day with ease; the urine amounts to three pints in twenty-four-hours; is amber colored and no sediment is found on standing a day. In health the urine does not have to be passed at night after retiring. A healthy person is free from all aches and pains of every kind. Many persons call themselves perfectly healthy yet suffer many aches and pains. A healthy person does not cough or expectorate nor is he obliged to blow his nose. The **pulse** of a healthy adult ranges from 70 to 80 a minute. Life insurance companies will insure persons with a pulse as low as 58 or as high as 88, provided all the other conditions are favorable; a person whose pulse is outside of this range when sitting still is not in perfect health. Fever and exertion of any kind will increase the frequency of the pulse. So will tobacco smoking. At birth the natural pulse is about 130 a minute, at two years about 100, at five years between 80 and 90, and gradually decreases in frequency until adult life is reached. In health the **temperature** of the body is 98½ degrees when taken by the thermometer in the mouth. A person whose temperature varies one degree from this figure is not in perfect health. If the temperature falls below 96 or rises above 106 death usually follows. There are rare exceptions to this rule.

What is Disease ? Any derangement of the mental or physical machinery is termed disease. Disturbances may be so slight as to be scarcely perceptible; again they may be so great as to affect every function of the body and mind.

Causes of Disease. The exciting causes of diseases are numerous, but the fundamental cause is unequal circulation. Heat expands and cold contracts. If one part of the body becomes cold there will be less blood in the cold part, and too much in some other part; that is a congestion of some other part. Every observing person knows the consequences of getting the feet damp and cold, or of sitting in a draft. Sitting quietly in one position for a long time with the mind active, disturbs the equilibrium of the circulation. An over-loaded stomach will also disturb circulation, so will a drink of ice water or a dish of ice cream. Errors of diet cause a large percentage of diseases; more than the average person imagines or the average physician recognizes. Contagious diseases are caused by microscopic germs. But they seem to make no progress until there is a disturbance of the circulation. It is certain, also, that they increase the disturbance of the circulation. A correction of a mental or physical derangement is a cure. Simply temporary relief is termed palliative. The distinction should be kept in mind.

Ways of Cure. Cures are made in many ways. By diversion of the thoughts, by change of climate, by change of diet, by mechanical and surgical means, by the application of electricity and by drugs. Drugs used to correct mental or physical derangement are medicines. From the beginning of history there have been numerous theories regarding the method of giving drugs. How drugs act is a question that has claimed the attention of the greatest minds in all ages. It would take volumes to recount the many theories that have been advanced. There is one theory, however, that was mentioned by Hippocrates before the Christian Era and elaborated by Samuel Hahnemann a century ago that has stood the test of time and has been demonstrated to be a natural law of cure. The following Latin phrase has been used to express this law; *similia similibus curantur*, liberally interpreted it means like cures like. According to this law that drug is given to a sick person which given to a well person produces symptoms similar to those which the sick person possesses. For instance, if you wish to determine the medicinal properties of a drug or plant of which you know nothing about, you would make a decoction of the plant and give it to a number of well persons and watch the effect it produced on them. If, after taking the drug for a time the majority of the persons were to have a throbbing headache, a flushed face and a sore throat on the right side with a constant tendency to swallow, we should rightfully conclude that the decoction had produced the symptoms, and when we came across a sick person with them we would give some of this decoction, but in diluted form as experience has shown to be best. Observation has shown that Belladonna produces the above set of symptoms; that it cures a sick person with these symptoms has been verified probably a million times. The medicinal uses of nearly a thousand drugs have been ascertained in this way. A collection of the symptoms produced by the various drugs and plants is called the **Homeopathic Materia Medica**. A person who is thoroughly familiar with the Materia Medica is well equipped to combat with most diseases. He has a rule by which he prescribes, that is as invariable as the law of gravitation. A person who once becomes familiar with the application of this law of cure will prefer it to all others. Like all other innovations and advances it has from time to time met with the bitterest and most stubborn opposition. Its author, Dr. Hahnemann, suffered the martyrdom that usually befalls every great discoverer and benefactor of the race. He was ridiculed, abused, ostracised and driven from place to place. Homeopathy is daily becoming more popular, its patrons are now numbered by millions. The more intelligent every where prefer it. Some fifteen thousand physicians in the United States alone practice it. Statistics gathered repeatedly from reliable sources show that the death rate is about one-half less under the Homeopathic treatment than it is under any other treatment. In other words, it has been demonstrated that a person who employs Homeopathic treatment has his chances of dying reduced fully fifty per cent. when compared with his chances under other methods of treatment. This is more than true in violent, contagious diseases, such as cholera, yellow fever, scarlet fever, typhoid, pneumonia, etc. During the recent cholera epidemic in Hamburg the death rate under Homeopathic treatment did not reach five per cent., while under other treatments the death rate was nearly fifty per cent. Experience has shown that when medicine is given according to the Homeopathic law, but a very small quantity is necessary to produce the desired effect. Instead of giving strong decoctions and tinctures Homeopathic physicians usually have their medicines diluted many times. Drugs diluted seem to act more quickly and there is no danger of the patient being poisoned by the crude drug, as has happened so often when drugs are given in accordance with other systems of medicines.

Homeopathic medicines generally used are diluted three times. Some are diluted many times. For instance, a drop of the tincture or crude drug is diluted in nine parts of alcohol. This mixture is labeled 1x. One drop of the 1x mixture mixed with nine drops of alcohol is called 2x preparation. One drop of the 2x mixed with nine of alcohol is called 3x dilution or potency. When the drug is a powder, sugar of milk is used instead of alcohol. The alcohol and sugar of milk are simply neutral vehicles, having no medicinal qualities. It is a strange fact that some drugs have greater medicinal force when greatly diluted than they do when in the crude form. Homeopathic medicines, as usually prepared, have no bad effect upon a well person. Children have been known to eat an entire bottle of Homeopathic pills and suffer no ill effects. This fact has been often used as an argument against Homeopathy, but it counts for nothing. Homeopathic medicine is intended to cure and not to kill. The old idea that medicine to be of any value must be bitter and disagreeable is absurd, and the relic of ignorance and barbarism. Every one knows that when our eyes are well and in their normal condition we suffer no inconvenience when we go out at midday into the brightest sunshine. But let our eyes be sore and inflamed; in other words, let them be sick, a single ray of sunlight will affect them. Likewise when every part of our mental and physical machinery is in perfect order, a whole bottle of Homeopathic medicine will not produce any perceptible effect, but let us be sick in any part and it requires but a single pellet, provided it be of the right kind, to affect us favorably.

While a thousand different drugs and plants have been studied and their medicinal uses determined, some thirty-five will cure the majority of the cases of sickness. As a rule but one drug should be given at a time. If the case is very sudden and acute the medicine may be repeated at short intervals, as often as fifteen minutes, but if the case is chronic and one of long standing, the doses should not be repeated so often; from one to six times a day. Some physicians, in such cases, repeat the medicine but once a week. Another rule observed by many physicians is not to repeat the dose as long as there are signs of improvement. In short they do not give the second dose until the first ceases to act.

Patent Medicines. If one understands Homeopathy he will appreciate the absurdity of some of the claims made for patent medicines. No two persons are exactly alike. In the same way no two cases of sickness are exactly alike. It is therefore absurd to expect what will help one will help another. The prescribing of the same patent medicine for a number of cases, when there is but a slight resemblance between any two cases, is simply guessing. A practical knowledge of the Homeopathic law will do more than anything else to do away with the now prevalent and often very injurious habit of using and prescribing patent medicines.

Opiates. There is a class of drugs known as opiates that are given to relieve pain or to produce sleep. They do not cure, but simply relieve for the time being. To give opiates is about as wise as it is to borrow money at usurious rate of interest. The principal and interest must be paid back sooner or later. A large class of physicians have the bad habit of giving opiates for every severe pain. They usually resort to opiates because they do not know what else to do to relieve their patient. A person who has a practical knowledge of the Homeopathic Materia Medica will rarely have occasion to resort to opiates. Homeopathic medicines not only relieve but they cure. They are curative, not simply palliative. Homeopathic medicine often relieves pain much quicker than any opiate. We have seen the most violent colic relieved within a few minutes by colocynth or aconite. The case was not only relieved, but cured. Persons without a practical knowledge of Homeopathy would have given an opiate and prolonged the sickness perhaps for many days, as is often the case.

Palliatives. Palliatives are drugs and means taken to give temporary relief. A person in the last stage of some incurable disease is often given some drug to give temporary relief. Opiates are the usual palliatives.

Prevention of Diseases. It is a trite saying that "An ounce of prevention is worth a pound of cure." The average person gives so little attention to the matter of preventing diseases that there is but little encouragement to spend much time on this all important subject. A hundred dollars to cure and not a cent to prevent. As we have already stated, a perfect circulation is the best preventive of disease. A person whose circulation is perfect cannot be sick. The best preventive against contagious diseases is pure blood. It is said that no germ can live in healthy blood. It is only when the blood becomes unhealthy that the germs of disease find a fertile soil and develop. We have already stated that errors of diet are a common cause of disease. More than half of all cases of sickness have their beginning in a deranged digestion. Attention to diet must be mentioned as the most important preventive. Lack of proper rest and proper exercise is another prolific source of disease. Over exertion and under exertion lead to the same results. When the system is tired disease more easily develops. Irregular hours of sleep is productive of much trouble. The average person requires eight hours of sleep, quiet, restful, refreshing sleep. Excesses, mental or physical, in any direction, are highly injurious. The bad effects may not be felt at the time, but sooner or later they will manifest themselves. This is specially true of the young, who always need a check upon their extravagance of physical energy. There is not a truer saying than "What we sow in our youth we shall reap in our age." In youth the seeds of decay are often sown. Parents and guardians cannot be too watchful over the habits of those under their care. Every physician of much experience knows that pernicious habits are often formed in youth, which undermine the health, mentally and physically.

PART I.

Description and Treatment of Diseases.

All diseases are divided into two general classes, namely: Local and constitutional. Those affections which are confined to a limited part of the body are classed as local, as for example, a felon. Those which affect the entire organism, such as typhoid fever, are classed as constitutional.

CONSTITUTIONAL DISEASES.

A large proportion of the constitutional diseases are infectious. An infectious disease is one that is caused by the presence of a certain specific germ in the organism. Infectious diseases are usually accompanied by fever. While probable yet it is not proven that all fevers are caused by infectious diseases.

FEVERS.

The most positive sign of a fever is a more or less enduring elevation of the temperature of the body above 98½ degrees. A fever is usually preceded by a period called incubation, during which there is a lassitude and indisposition on the part of the patient. This is followed by a chill or chilly sensation, after which there is a rise of temperature with an increase of the frequency of the pulse. There is often pain in the head, back and limbs, also great restlessness. If the fever is very high delirium may occur. While all fevers have certain features in common yet there are differences and peculiarities which enable us to distinguish three classes of fevers. Those in which the fever is *continued* without interruption from the beginning to the end of the attack, as for example, typhoid fever. Those which have periods of complete intermission of the fever for a day or two, and then another rise for a similar period. These are called *periodical* fevers. The third class embraces those fevers which are distinguished by a rash or an eruption upon the skin. This class is designated as the *eruptive* fevers.

ERUPTIVE FEVERS.

There are three well defined stages of eruptive fevers. First, the stage of invasion; dating from the first disturbance of the health to the appearance of the eruption. The second, the eruptive stage, which dates from the beginning of the eruption until its disappearance. Third, the stage of desquamation, or of the peeling off.

The eruptive fevers include small-pox, measles, scarlet fever and chicken-pox. It is important to remember that the eruption of chicken-pox breaks out during the first day of sickness; scarlet fever during the second day; small-pox during the third, while the eruption of measles does not make its appearance until the fourth day of the sickness. It will also aid in determining the nature of the disease; if it is remembered that small-pox begins with a very severe chill; that scarlet fever is usually accompanied by a sore throat, and that a cough is always a prominent symptom in measles. It will be of advantage to note that the eruption of small-pox appears first about the mouth and chin; that of chicken-pox is first seen upon the body and limbs; that of measles behind the ears and on the face; and that the first appearance of the scarlet fever eruption is upon the neck and chest.

CHICKEN-POX.

This is the mildest of the eruptive diseases, being rarely if ever fatal. It is confined to children. It is infectious; also contag'ous.

Symptoms.—The appearance of the eruption is generally preceded by slight constitutional disturbances for about twenty-four hours. There is some fever; possibly, nausea and vomiting. The rash usually appears first on the body, and afterwards on the face and head. It is easily distinguished from the eruption of small-pox, by the fact that it is *from the first* composed of *vesicles* (blisters), and not of hard *papules* (pimples). On the fifth or sixth day the vesicles begin to dry; by this time they may be as large as small peas, and are surrounded by a broad, red margin. They soon scab and fall off, rarely leaving scars. Not infrequently a second crop of vesicles appears during the first three days. Chicken-pox manifests itself from ten to fifteen days after exposure.

Treatment.—Chicken-pox rarely requires any special treatment. Good nursing and a little attention to diet will be, as a rule, all that is needed. In case of considerable fever, with restlessness, **Aconite** may be given. Should there be a sore throat, a flushed face and starting during sleep, give **Belladonna.** In case of a watery discharge from the eyes and nose, **Pulsatilla** will be indicated.

SCARLET FEVER.

This fever derives its name from the scarlet eruption that is always present in a typical case. In some cases the eruption is so slight as to be scarcely perceptible. Attacks vary in intensity from a mild affection to one of the most malignant of diseases. Physicians sometimes distinguish three varieties. But the only difference between them is the degree of severity. A mild case may give the contagion to another who will have the disease in the severest form. In order to contract scarlet fever one must come within a few feet of the patient. Measles and whooping cough may be taken when one is at a considerable distance. A number of instances are recorded where clothing and other articles used about a scarlet fever patient have been packed into a trunk and months afterwards opened in the house of some distant family where there were children and soon afterwards some of the children have had the disease. It is recorded that a mother who lost her only child with scarlet fever packed its toys away. In course of time she became the mother of another child, and when it became old enough to appreciate toys the playthings of the former child were unpacked and soon afterwards it also had the disease. The importance of destroying or disinfecting all articles that have been about a scarlet fever patient is obvious. In ninety per cent. of all cases of scarlet fever the patient is under ten years of age. We have treated a few cases where the patients were between twenty and thirty years. It rarely attacks children under one year of age. One child may have a very severe attack, while another in the same family may have the disease in the mildest form.

As soon as a case of scarlet fever is discovered in a family of children the case should be isolated by confining it to one room and keeping all others out   The rest of the children should be given **Belladonna 3x** four times a day. We have never seen a second severe case of scarlet fever occur in the same family when this course was pursued. Even when the sick and well were not separated we have never seen another member of the family have the disease in any but the lightest form.

Scarlet fever is contagious from the first day of the attack until the peeling off stage is completed. It has been quite conclusively shown that the disease is infectious; in other words a germ disease. It may be carried in the clothing of the physician or nurse; and even by letters written in the sick room. It has been demonstrated that the fumes of sulphur do not readily kill these germs. One of the best and most agreeable disinfectants that can be used in the room during the progress of the disease is prepared as follows: One ounce of carbolic acid, one ounce of the oil of eucalyptus and six ounces of the spirits of turpentine are mixed together. Two tablespoonfuls of the mixture are put into a quart of water and kept simmering over an oil or gas stove. The patient may be disinfected and made more comfortable by rubbing the entire surface of the body several times a day with an ointment made by mixing together one drachm of carbolic acid, one drahm of eucalyptus oil and seven ounces of olive oil. The room occupied by a scarlet fever patient should be large and well ventilated. During the eruptive stage the temperature of the room should be 68 degrees. After the peeling off stage begins it should be raised to 73. The patient should be guarded against all exposure and kept in bed ten or twelve days.

Symptoms.—The period of incubation, that is the interval between exposure and the first manifestation of the disease, varies from three to twelve days. The period is usually shorter that that of other eruptive diseases. The onset is usually sudden. It may be preceded by a very slight indisposition. A chill is rare, but vomiting and, in young children, convulsions are common. The fever may be intense, rising rapidly and reaching 104 or 105 degrees the first day, causing headache and delirium. The skin is unusually dry and imparts a peculiar burning sensation when the palm of the hand is placed in contact with it. Dryness and soreness of the throat on swallowing are common symptoms. The inside of the throat is as a rule unnaturally red and the glands at the angles of the jaw swollen. The rash usually appears the second day in the form of scattered red points on a deep flush. It appears on the neck and chest first. It spreads so rapidly that by the evening of the second day it may have covered the entire body. In marked, typical cases the rash at its height has a vivid scarlet hue, distinct and unlike that seen in any other disease. The tongue in many cases is firey red with raised papillae and is described as the "strawberry tongue." The rash usually remains out from four to six days.

Desquamation.—About the sixth day the rash begins to fade and during the succeeding days the surface of the skin is thrown off in the form of bran like scales. Sometimes, however, large pieces of the skin may come off. We have seen pieces covering a whole finger or the greater part of the palm or heel shed at one time. The peeling off process continues from one to two weeks.

Between the second and third week of the disease, when convalescence seems to be progressing finely, the kidneys will sometimes show signs of inflammation. Little or no urine will be passed. Or there will be a frequent desire, but only a small quantity of black, smoky urine voided. The face and eye lids will be puffed.

It is a serious complication and may follow the mildest attack. It causes almost as many deaths as occur during the earlier stage of the disease. The importance of careful nursing and a simple diet until after the third week, is apparent. Another serious trouble which sometimes follows scarlet fever is inflammation and suppuration of the ear with deafness. Chronic weakness of the eyes have also been caused by scarlet fever.

Treatment.—It should be emphasized right here that the foregoing complications are of very rare occurrence in cases treated Homeopathically. Statistics gathered from many reliable sources show that Homeopathic physicians have a death rate from this disease less than half as great as that of other physicians.

When medicines fail to control the high fever and congestion to the head, the patient may be wrapped in a blanket wrung out of water at the temperature of the room. The process may be repeated until the temperature is decidedly lowered. If an ice cap cannot be procured, a cloth wrung out of the coldest water should be applied to the head and reapplied as often as it gets warm.

Diet.—During this, as in all other fevers, the less food taken the better. Milk and water in equal parts taken warm is sufficient. Plenty of cool water may be given. If the diet is carefully guarded kidney complications are less likely to occur.

Belladonna.—In eighty per cent. of all cases, the only remedy required. Eruption perfectly smooth and bright scarlet red. Flushed face. Head hot. Delirium. Throbbing at sides of neck and temples. Starts and jumps while asleep.

Bryonia.—The eruption does not come out fully or suddenly disappears. Lungs or brain affected.

Arsenicum.—The eruption delays or grows suddenly pale

with rapid prostration. Putrid sore throat. Great anguish and extreme restlessness. Intense thirst. Wheezing respiration. Foul diarrhœa.

Rhus Tox.—Rash is dark colored and itches violently. Drowsy or delirious. Restless. The eyes have the appearance of one intoxicated. Nose-bleed at night. Rheumatism. The eruption has a rough appearance.

Lachesis.—Marked swelling of the glands of the neck. Worse on the left side.

Sulphur.—Eruption growing purple. Brain symptoms. Nose dry. Mouth and throat so dry cannot speak plainly. Stupor. Violent itching. Child jumps and screams.

MEASLES.

Measles is not so fatal a disease as scarlet fever. But it is often followed by weaknesses that remain and disturb the health for years. The writer suffered from bronchitis for fifteen years as a result of measles improperly treated. We have seen a number of persons whose eyes had been weak years after an attack of measles. Here again we must call attention to the fact that in measles as well as in scarlet fever complications rarely follow homeopathic treatment of the disease. It is a germ disease. But the germs are unlike those of scarlet fever and diphtheria, in that they do not cling to the clothing, bedding, articles of furniture and walls of the room, or things handled by the patient. Like those of whooping cough, they seem to float in the air and not to adhere to anything. For this reason it cannot be carried by nurses and physicians, as scarlet fever and diphtheria may be. For the same reason it cannot be isolated and confined, as those diseases may be. When a case occurs in a family, school or asylum, the disease usually attacks all the inmates that have not previously had it.

A thorough airing of the apartments which have been occupied by a case of measles and a washing of the bedding, clothing and furniture will be sufficient precautions against the disease for the next occupant of the room. The disease usually attacks children, but no age is exempt from it. It is usually more severe in adults and persons of a dark complexion. The disease rarely occurs a second time in the same person.

Symptoms.—Measles usually manifests itself about ten days after exposure. The period of incubation, however, may be longer or shorter. It begins as a feverish cold. There are shiverings, sneezing, running of the nose, redness and watering of the eyes. Later a severe cough and bronchial catarrh, with constriction of the chest.

There may be nausea, vomiting, headache and wandering pains. Nose bleed, croup and convulsions may occur. Before the eruption appears the disease may be mistaken for a number of other complaints. On the fourth day the rash usually appears, first behind the ears, on the temples and on the forehead, in the form of small red pimples, which increase in size and spread over the neck and chest. When the eruption is well out the face is swollen with red blotches. Sometimes the skin feels as if there were shot just beneath the surface. It requires about four days from the first appearance of the eruption for it to spread over the entire body. From any given part the rash begins to fade in thirty-six hours from the time it appeared on that part. The eruption may be suppressed from taking cold, by indiscretion in eating and by taking purgatives. A suppression of the eruption is a serious complication and needs prompt treatment. On the fourth day of the rash the fever subsides and the rash fades. The skin does not peel off in large flakes as in scarlet fever, but in very fine dust or bran like scales. The most important sequel of measles is some weakness of the lungs. On account of the frequent occurrence of consumption after measles it ranks third among eruptive diseases, in comparing the death rate.

Treatment.—During an attack of measles the patient should be kept in a darkened room and not allowed to use the eyes. Should the eruption be tardy or delayed in coming out the warm pack will be of value. Measles without complications require but little treatment. Precautions against taking cold are most important.

Aconite.—First stage. Fever, high; chest, oppressed. Restless. Skin hot and dry. Pulse full and quick. Great thirst.

Arsenicum.—Severe case. Delirious or stupid. Rash suppressed. Itching of skin. Craves cold drinks. Urine suppressed or scanty. Face bloated. Lips parched. Very weak. Pale. Worse about one o'clock at night

Bryonia.—Eruption does not appear, or driven in by cold. Severe cough. Congestion to lungs, with sharp, sticking pains. Difficult breathing. Sitting up causes nausea.

Pulsatilla.—Useful in first stage, or during any stage when the catarrh is profuse. Thick, yellow discharge from nose. Worse toward evening. Stomach deranged. Craves fresh air. Rattling of phlegm in chest. Diarrhœa following suppressed rash. Mucous discharges. Useful in developing the rash. Most useful remedy.

Phosphorus.—Tightness across the chest; violent and exhausting cough. Stitching pains; worse with every breath.

Sulphur.—Useful in the beginning to bring out rash and also for the after effects of the disease. Brings about reaction.

SMALL-POX.

This disease was formerly the dread and scourge of nations, but now it is an infrequent and a comparatively harmless visitor. The wonderful change has been brought about by vaccination, the discovery of Jenner in 1798. It is said that in the year 1837 small-pox attacked the Mandan Indians and within twelve months, out of a population of 150,000 only twenty-seven remained. Small-pox is just as destructive to-day as ever where vaccination is not enforced. It has been well nigh stamped out of all civilized countries. No age is exempt from small-pox, but the younger the person the more severe the attack and greater the death rate. One attack usually prevents a second. In Chicago no child is allowed to enter the public schools without being vaccinated. The rule should be universal. Every person should be vaccinated. After exposure to the disease one should lose no time in being vaccinated. If vaccination be done within twenty-four hours after exposure it will either entirely prevent or greatly modify the disease. The longer it is delayed the less likely it is to do either.

Symptoms.—In adults a severe chill and in children a convulsion are the first pronounced symptoms. The chill may be repeated. An intense frontal headache, severe pains across the middle of the back and vomiting are rarely absent. The pains and chill are more violent in this than in any other eruptive fever. Their violence alone, during an epidemic of small-pox, would warrant a diagnosis of that disease. The temperature may reach 104 degrees the first day and continue gradually to rise during the next two days. The face is flushed. There may be delirium. The eyes are bright and clear. The skin is usually dry, but there may be profuse sweat. The strongest may, within twenty-four hours after the ushering in of a chill, be unable to get out of bed.

The severity of the first symptoms bears no relation to the severity of the attack. After the fever has continued three full days the eruption will show itself first on the forehead near the hair or about the mouth and chin; also on the wrists. The extension of the rash over the entire body requires two or three days longer. With the appearance of the eruption the fever and all other symptoms subside. The rash at first consists of small red spots, the size of a pin-head. They gradually increase in size and become elevated and hard, having the feel of shot under the skin. As the pimples enlarge a depression is, as a rule, formed in the center of the summit. From the sixth to the eighth day after the first appearance of the eruption the pimples fill with pus, that is maturate or suppurate. The skin about them becomes greatly swollen; the whole face swells beyond recognition, closing the eyes. The hands and feet are swollen until they look like round balls. The itching at this stage is unbearable and the odor sickening. It is during this stage that the most deaths occur. By the ninth day the process of suppuration has reached its height and the pimples or pustules either rupture or begin to dry up. About the fourteenth day the scabs fall off. About the eighth or ninth day, when the process of suppuration is at its highest, there is a secondary fever, beginning with a chill, which rises even higher than the initial fever. There are varieties of small-pox, but the chief difference is the degree of severity.

Varioloid is a mild form of small-pox, occurring in those who have been vaccinated or have had the disease. It is capable of communicating the genuine disease.

Treatment.—In the character of its contagiousness small-pox is very much like scarlet fever. Many of the directions given for isolating and disinfecting a case of the latter disease will apply to one of the former. It is important that the patient be placed in a large, well ventilated room as remote as possible from the other members of the family, and not more than one person or two at most, be allowed to attend or visit him. All unnecessary articles of furniture, curtains and carpets should be removed from the room. The patient's hair should be cut short and all flannel clothing removed. Every effort should be made to keep the patient and his bedding clean. When matter forms in the pimples the room should be darkened.

The itching may be relieved by applying carbolized vaseline or vaseline with a little iodoform mixed in it. Some have found that a better way to relieve the itching is to apply lint wrung out of cold water. Some antiseptic, such as carbolic acid or bichloride of mercury, may be added to the water. Cold water, no doubt, has a very soothing and beneficial effect. Great precaution should be taken to protect the eyes by frequent washing.

As for internal remedies the best and most recent old school medical authorities confess that they know of no drug that will cut short or particularly modify an attack of small-pox. But when we turn to our Homeopathic authorities we do not find so much skepticism. There are a number of Homeopathic remedies that are very useful in this dreaded disease.

Tartar Emetic.—The most useful remedy in small-pox. Should be given from the first to the last of the attack. Especially valuable during the eruptive stage. It lessens the severity of the disease. Prevents pitting in most cases.

Arsenicum.—Useful in the latter part of the attack when there is great prostration, thirst and nausea; when the eruption has a livid appearance. Odor very offensive.

Aconite and **Belladonna** are likely to be indicated in the earlier part of the attack when the fever and the congestion of the brain are prominent symptoms.

Mercurius, Rhus Tox, Baptisia Pulsatilla, Apis or Sulphur may be indicated during the course of the disease. The special symptoms for giving them may be determined by a careful study of the Materia Medica, Part II.

DIPHTHERIA.

Whether this disease is a local or a constitutional affection at the beginning of the attack is a question that has been, and is still very much discussed. That it is constitutional in a later stage is conceded by all. The particular germ that causes the disease has been discovered and is easily distinguished from all other germs. Diphtheria has prevailed from the earliest times. It is not peculiar to any climate or any time of the year. It is usually more prevalent in the spring and autumn. It generally affects children, especially between two and five years, but it is not uncommon among adults. It occurs more frequently among the poor, but the well-to-do families do not escape it. One attack does not prevent a second. It is not confined to cities. In cities, however, the disease seems to be on the increase. There is a general belief that there is some connection between diphtheria and defective drainage, but just what the relation is, has not yet been clearly established. It has been suggested that the poor drainage may cause sore throat and the sore throat afford a fertile soil for the diphtheritic germ

It is certain that exposure to cold and the resultant disturbance of the circulation favors the development of the disease. We have laid it down as a fundamental proposition derived from our personal observation that a disturbance of the circulation, a congestion to some part, is a prime essential before any germ disease can develop.

In support of this view we find that persons who have enlarged tonsils and catarrh of the throat are more susceptible to diphtheria than those who are not thus affected. It requires from two to fourteen days after exposure for the disease to show itself. The germs may lie dormant for months. They have been preserved in a piece of dry cloth five months. It is plain, therefore, that great care should be exercised by those in charge of a case of diphtheria. The same precautions given for the isolation of a scarlet fever patient should be observed. Even greater care should be taken, for of all infectious diseases now common, it is the most to be dreaded. The patient's room should be large, airy, and if possible, at the top of the house. If the room has a fire-place, so much the better. Carpets, rugs, curtains, pictures and all unnecessary furniture should be removed. A sheet, kept wet with some disinfecting solution, should be hung outside of the door. The special attendants should be the only persons allowed in the room. Dishes, towels, clothing, bedding and other articles used in the room should be kept there and not allowed to be carried through the house and used elsewhere. Dishes and like utensils should be washed in the patient's room or in some room not used by other members of the family. Soiled clothes should be soaked in a disinfecting solution or in boiling water for several hours before being taken from the room. All discharges from the patient should be received into china or glass vessels containing a solution of bichloride of mercury in the proportion of 1 to 5000. Cats, dogs, birds and other household pets should be kept out of the room. Even flies should be kept out, for they too have been supposed to carry infection. The plumbing and drains should be carefully examined and defects promptly repaired. Articles of food should not be left exposed in the room. Milk is especially likely to absorb impurities.

All discharges from the mouth, nose and throat of a diphtheritic patient are loaded with germs. During the examination or treatment of the throat it has often happened that the patient coughed into the face of the physician and in this way communicated the disease. In making examinations of cases of this kind the physician should tie a handkerchief over his face, covering his nose and mouth. The handkerchief should afterwards be disinfected. It is related that a few months ago some flowers from the coffin of a child who had died of diphtheria were afterwards thrown away and picked up by some children passing along. They took the disease and communicated it to the physician who treated them. It proved fatal in his case. Physicians, while treating diphtheria, have taken blood poisoning through a wound on the hand. The disinfecting mixture given in the chapter on scarlet fever should be kept simmering on an oil stove in the room.

Symptoms.—These vary greatly. The onset may be sudden or it may be slow and insidious. In one case the constitutional symptoms may be noticed first, in another the attention is first directed to the local. The constitutional symptoms may begin with a severe chill or there may be only chilly sensations. Children may have convulsions. There is usually a pain in the head, neck, back and limbs. As a rule the fever in diphtheria rises more slowly than in any other infectious disease. The temperature may run high in some cases while in others it may attain no great elevation, even though they are severe cases. In most febrile diseases the temperature is a better criterion than the pulse by which to determine the severity of the disease. But in diphtheria the pulse is more likely to be the better guide.

The local symptoms begin with a sense of dryness and prick101ng in the throat. Stiffness and swelling at the angles of the jaw soon follow; also pain on swallowing. White patches scattered over the tonsils appear a few hours later. These rapidly spread and run together, forming one continuous membrane upon the tonsils and adjacent parts. The membrane now becomes a dirty grey and later may become black. If a piece of it be scraped off a raw, bleeding surface will be found. The bleeding is considered one of the reliable signs of diphtheria. If the membrane is easily wiped off and no bleeding follows the probabilities are that the case is not one of diphtheria. If, however, there should be swelling on the outside of the throat at the angles of the jaw, along with the patches on the inside, the chances are ten to one that the case is diphtheritic. If a microscopical examination of some of the substance that composes a patch reveals the presence of the specific germs of diphtheria no further evidence is necessary. Such an examination, however, can only be made by an expert microscopist. In diphtheria the tongue is usually clean, while in tonsillitis it is heavily coated.

If albumen be found in the urine of a case of suspected diphtheria it confirms the suspicions. Any physician or druggist can make the test for albumen within a few minutes, by simply boiling a little of the urine in a test tube over an alcohol lamp and then adding a few drops of nitric acid. If a milky deposit remains, albumen is present.

The membrane is at first seen on one tonsil, later it appears on the other and may extend to the palate, forward to the roof of the mouth, into the ear, upward into the nose, or downward into the windpipe. When the disease extends downward it is called diphtheritic or membranous croup. The chances of recovery are then greatly lessened.

The signs that indicate that the membrane is extending downward into the trachea is an increasing hoarseness and a croupy cough, with difficult breathing. When these symptoms become prominent and suffocation threatens, tracheotomy or intubation is required. The first consists in making an opening into the windpipe through the skin at a point just below the prominence called 'Adam's apple,' and inserting a curved silver tube. Intubation is a later operation, which requires no cutting and is performed by inserting a gold-plated tube down the windpipe through the mouth. Though having the advantage of being bloodless, it has the disadvantage of not allowing as much air to enter the lungs as tracheotomy does. Life is saved in about one-fourth of the cases in which these operations are performed.

Diphtheria runs a very rapid course. Death or convalescence usually takes place within a week. There may be complications and after effects that will remain a long time. Paralysis of various muscles may occur. Some of the muscles of the throat are most frequently affected, indicated by difficulty in swallowing. For instance in drinking, the water often comes out of the nose. Some of the muscles of the legs are often affected, indicated by an inability or an awkwardness in walking. Paralysis following diphtheria yields readily, as a rule, to homeopathic medicines. Paralysis following an acute attack of sore throat is good evidence that the throat trouble was diphtheritic, even if there were no other signs of diphtheria.

Paralysis occur two or three weeks after the active symptoms of the disease have disappeared. Paralysis of the heart may occur when the patient seems to be out of all danger. As a rule, the older the patient the more chances of recovery. The eminent old school authority, Mackenzie, lays it down as a rule that one-third of all the typical cases of diphtheria prove fatal. But the death rate under homeopathic treatment is not nearly so great. Statistics gathered recently in the city of Brooklyn show that the homeopathic loss from this disease is about 60 per cent. less than that from the old school treatment.

Treatment.—Very few physicians can boast of uniform success in the treatment of diphtheria. As a rule they will very cheerfully resign the case to the next doctor. The experience of many is illustrated by the following story: A stranger, on arriving in a western town which had but two hotels, asked a street corner loafer to tell him which was the better hotel. The loafer giving his cud of tobacco an extra roll and relieving himself of a mouthful of tobacco juice, replied, "Stranger, no matter to which hotel you go, you will be "durned" sorry in the morning that you did not go to the other." Likewise, it frequently happens that in treating diphtheria, whatever remedy the physician gives he is afterwards sorry that he did not give the other medicine.

The rapid loss of strength and the great exhaustion are striking features of diphtheria. All concede the necessity of maintaining the strength. But how to do this, is the question. Many insist on forced feeding of rich concentrated foods; predigested meat juice, bovinine, peptonized milk, raw eggs, beet tea slightly thickened with rice or pearl barley, arrow root or sago, with sherry or port, eggs beaten up with milk or in brandy with water or sugar, ice cream. They insist that the food shall be given regularly during the night as well as during the day; every four or six hours. The patient with this disease, as a rule, stubbornly refuses food. It may be partly from loss of appetite, but no doubt principally because of the discomfort experienced on swallowing. Spraying the throat with a four per cent. solution of cocaine renders swallowing easier. In its poisonous effects upon the blood diphtheria in some way resembles typhoid. If there is one thing upon which we have a positive opinion it is that the less food given to a typhoid fever patient the better. We have found that in typhoid we get the best results when we give no food whatever during the first week of the disease. Others maintain that milk, with lime water in it, is sufficient nourishment for a diphtheritic patient. Raw milk favors the development of germs. The lime water destroys this quality of the milk and it is therefore essential that a tablespoonful of lime water be added to every cupful of milk.

If no food can be got into the stomach through the mouth it should be injected into the bowels every six hours. That brandy should be given when there is danger of heart failure is generally conceded. We have recently seen two cases, age four years, successfully "tided" over the danger of heart failure by giving one teaspoonful of brandy every hour day and night. We feel morally certain that they would have proved fatal had not the brandy been given. It is an established fact that it is well nigh impossible to intoxicate a person who has diphtheria. The danger, therefore, is not in giving too much brandy, but in giving too little. It is a clear case of treating poison with poison. There is a danger of being misled by the false stimulation. Extra vigilance is therefore required when alcoholic stimulants are given. It has seemed to us that their use prolonged convalescence. Patients should not be allowed to sit up longer than is absolutely necessary, as sitting taxes the heart more than lying. A patient threatened with heart failure should have the head lower than the body. Recently a little patient under our care during convalescence unexpectedly showed signs of heart failure. No one was present except the trained nurse, but she was equal to the emergency. On seeing the sudden blanching of the face and on failing to detect the pulse, she stood the child upon its head. In a few moments more she had put a teaspoonful of brandy into its mouth. The child is alive and well to-day. The watchfulness and prompt action of the nurse no doubt saved its life from heart failure.

Local Remedies.—Like everything else pertaining to diphtheria, the local treatment varies from absolutely no treatment whatever to the most violent and heroic measures. The advocates of both extremes have their successes and their failures. Alcohol and water in equal parts is a good gargle for patients old enough to use it. For younger patients it may be used as a spray in proportion, 1 to 6. Two or three grains of permanganate of potash in a glass of water make a pink gargle that is frequently used and has much real merit. Per oxide of hydrogen diluted one half with water, is also an excellent spray. A mixture of spirits of pepermint 10 parts, tannic acid 30 parts, mucilage of gum 100, painted on the tonsils and adjacent parts with a brush or thrown into the the throat by a small syringe, has given excellent satisfaction in many cases. It is quite effectual in removing the patches. A few minutes after its use the patient invariably feels better. A spray or gargle of the bi-chloride of mercury, 1 to 5,000, has given good results. Nurses taking care of diphtheria cases often use this gargle to protect themselves from the disease. Care should be taken that it is not used in too strong a solution, as we recently saw a horrible case of mercurial poisoning follow its use.

Constitutional Treatment.—Many hold to the theory that there must be some deviation from perfect health before diphtheria or any other infectious disease can attack a person. There are surely many facts to support such a theory. If the theory is correct then local treatment is only secondary, while the constitutional treatment is of prime importance. This is the view held by the best homeopathic physicians.

Aconite.—Useful for the fever in case the onset is sudden.

Apis.—Mouth and throat bright red and glossy, as if varnished. Pain in ears on swallowing. Paralysis of throat following diphtheria. Not much fever. No thirst. Great prostration from beginning. Face and neck puffy. Inside of throat has a puffy appearance. Palate looks like a little bag filled with water. Patches look like a piece of chamois skin. Worse on the right side. Difficult breathing. Urine scanty. Said to prevent diphtheria.

Arsenicum.—Advanced stage of blood poisoning. Membrane dark. Constant desire for cold drinks, but can take little. Worse about midnight. Pinched and deathly look.

Baptisia.—No pain on swallowing. Can swallow liquids only. Least solid food gags. Prostration great. Stupid, besotted expression. Typhoid condition. Valuable remedy for the blood poisoning.

Belladonna.—Useful only at beginning. Fever high. Throat deep red. Very difficult swallowing. Neck stiff. Glands swollen. Throat dry. Drowsy, but can't sleep. Starts in sleep.

Kali Bichro.—Hoarse, croupy cough. Membrane looking pearly and extending downward. Expectorations, stringy, frequently blood streaked. Much swelling, but little redness.

Lachesis.—Patient complains of being worse than he appears. Patches begin on the left side and spread to the right. Neck sensitive to the slightest touch. Can bear nothing tight about the neck. Throat purplish. Feeling of a lump in the throat, or as if a crumb of bread had lodged there. More difficult to swallow liquids than solids. Throat painful on bending head back. Pain in throat extends to ears. Much phlegm, with painful hawking. Worse from hot drinks.

Lycopodium.—Begins on the right side and extends to the left. Feeling of contraction of throat, as if a ball rose from below. Chronic enlargement of tonsils. Odor foul. Everything tastes sour. Red sand in urine. Rumbling sensation in stomach and bowels. Worse from 4 to 8 p. m.

Liquor Calcis Chlorinatæ.—May be procured at any drug store. Put from 5 to 15 drops into half a glass of water. Give a teaspoonful at intervals of fifteen minutes to six hours. Indicated when there is great swelling of glands and a horribly foul odor. Belladonna antidotes it.

Mercurius Cor.—Patches cover entire throat; tonsils, palate, roof of mouth and back of throat. High fever. Lips dry, brown, cracked and bleeding. Saliva offensive. Eyes watery and sore. Burning discharges. Throat burns.

Nitric Acid.—When Mercurius fails to reduce swelling of glands. Have seen it rapidly reduce swollen glands that remained after disappearance of all symptoms from the inside of the throat.

Sulphur.—Powdered sulphur blown into the throat is a common remedy and believed to have a good deal of virtue.

Chlorate of Potash.—May be procured at any drug store. Five grains put into half a glass of water and given every four hours is claimed to be both a preventive and a curative of diphtheria. The dose for an infant under two years is one teaspoonful; children from two to six years, two teaspoonsful; older children, three teaspoonsful. For other remedies study Part II.

TYPHOID FEVER.

Excepting malarial, Typhoid is the most common of all fevers. It may be developed in any country or in any climate during any time of the year. It occurs, however, more frequently in the temperate zones and during the months of August, September and October. It prevails most in hot, dry seasons. It is found in the rural districts as well as in the cities. The majority of cases occur in robust persons between the ages of fifteen and twenty-four. It is rarely met in infants and persons over sixty. A specific germ is always found with Typhoid and it is therefore classed with the infectious diseases. It is but slightly contagious compared with the eruptive fevers. The germ peculiar to typhoid is found in the lymphoid tissues of the intestines, in the mesenteric glands, in the spleen and in the liver. It will be noticed that all these locations are below the diaphragm; that is, in the abdomen. It will be remembered that the germs of diphtheria are found only in the throat and nowhere else. The post mortem examination of those who have died of the disease shows this. The blood poisoning of diphtheria cannot, therefore, be from the germ direct, but must be due to some product of the germ. The resemblance of the blood poisoning in the two diseases has been noticed. While the local expression of diphtheria is in the throat that of typhoid is in that part of the intestines lying just above the right groin. This accounts for the fact that we find in almost every case of typhoid tenderness in that region.

The common vehicles of the typhoid infection are water, air, soiled linen of typhoid patients and the hands of the nurses. But it is believed that in ninety-nine times out of a hundred it is conveyed by the drinking water. The city of Geneva receives its drinking water from two rivers. It has been observed that all the cases of typhoid in that city drink the water from one river, while those who drink from the other source never have the disease.

The drinking water of Paris is derived from a number of sources. In dry seasons certain portions of the city are obliged to be supplied from a particular canal. It has been repeatedly noticed that within about two weeks after the water is turned on the number of typhoid patients in the district supplied by the canal increase three or four hundred per cent. During the winter of 1885, at Plymouth, Pa., a solitary case of typhoid fever occurred above the town on the bank of a river which supplied the drinking water. The discharges from the patient for several weeks were thrown out upon the snow without being disinfected. March 25th a thaw and rain melted the snow and it ran down the bank into the river. Exactly fourteen days later an epidemic of typhoid developed, amounting to 1,200 cases in that city of a population of only 8000. More than one hundred of the cases proved fatal. The cities of Geneva, Paris and Plymouth afford us a double lesson. First, that the water readily conveys the infection, and, second, that to disinfect every discharge from a typhoid patient is of the utmost importance; not to do so is criminal negligence. A solution of bi-chloride of mercury, 1 to 1000, will destroy typhoid germs. A solution of carbolic acid, 1 to 100, will also destroy them. Both are open to objections; the first is a dangerous poison, besides destructive to plumbing; the latter acts slowly, requiring several hours.

The only everywhere practical and thoroughly satisfactory disinfectant for the discharges from a typhoid patient is lime, used strong enough to make a "white-wash." All linen from a typhoid patient should be burned, or boiled for several hours. The nurse and physician should wash their hands with soap and water and afterwards rinse them in a solution of bi-chloride of mercury in proportion of one to a thousand. It should always be remembered that this solution of corrosive sublimate in such a strength is highly poisonous taken internally. Boil drinking water before using.

Symptoms.—The onset of typhoid fever is gradual and insidious. In this respect it is decidedly different from the eruptive fevers and most of the infectious diseases. The disease commences so imperceptibly that the majority of typhoid patients are unable to fix definitely the date their illness begun. It is, therefore, impossible to determine the exact period of incubation of typhoid. The average duration is supposed to be from three to ten days.

During the preliminary stage of the disease the patient usually continues at his work, yet he is conscious that he is not exactly well. Chilly sensations, shivering and perhaps a pronounced chill may occur. These may be repeated, especially the chilly sensations at irregular intervals. There is usually frontal headache and the mental faculties seem a little cloudy. The patient is unable to concentrate his thoughts with the usual vigor; feels generally languid and prostrated. Loss of appetite, nausea and even vomiting may occur. There is generally a looseness of the bowels. Nose bleed without any apparent cause is not an uncommon symptom. After these symptoms have been present for perhaps a week the individual will be forced to give up his occupation and go to bed. During the first few days there is, perhaps, a persistent, dull red flushing of the face. By the time he takes to his bed there is a lack of expression, a listlessness and even a stupidity that is quite noticeable to the most casual observer. A person coming down with typhoid may look and act like one somewhat deranged. They often will take no notice of what is said to them until they are repeatedly addressed and then perhaps their answer will be slow and disconnected. The unnatural redness of the skin of the face, arm and abdomen will disappear upon pressure with the tip of the finger, but on taking the finger away it will regain the color in a sluggish way never seen in health.

During the first week in bed, the patient, if not too stupid, will complain of considerable pain in the head. There may be insomnia during this period. Sometimes the mind will be apparently clear during the day, but at night there will be talking in the sleep and is confused on awakening. The mild delirium usually appears about the second week. There is, perhaps, a low muttering In many cases there will be attempts to get out of bed. Occasionally the patient gets boisterous when restrained. It should be borne in mind that no reliance can be placed in what the patient at this stage of the disease says. Their statements are unreliable. After recovery they will not remember what they said or what occurred. As soon as delirium manifests itself the patient should be constantly watched; should never be left alone even for a minute, for it has frequently happened that the patient got up, fell out the window or wandered away. Besides this, it is important that after the typhoid patient has once taken to his bed, that he should be kept there. Every time he rises is positively injurious. Absolute rest of the bowels in every way is a prime essential to the successful treatment of the disease.

Along with the delirium there will be an utter indifference to everything. The patient will not ask for food or drink though the mouth may be dry and parched. The nurse should not neglect to give the patient plenty of cool water, at regular intervals. The hearing is frequently affected and sometimes the sight. The patient will lie listless in one position in the bed until the skin becomes sore and bed-sores form if the nurse is not watchful, to bathe and rub dry the reddened places with a solution of tannic acid or arnica, or the two preparations mixed is even better than either singly. It should be noted that the patient often appears to be sleeping when he is not. He is easily aroused, but at once lapses back into semi-unconsciousness. In fact the loss of sleep is a source of the great nervous exhaustion. Another symptom that will be noted at this stage is a twitching of the tendons at the wrists. At times it will be so frequent as to render it difficult to take the pulse. There may be twitchings of other muscles. The twitchings indicate somewhat the severity of the attack. During second week dark brown matter accumulates on the teeth called sordes.

An accurate record of the temperature taken at six a. m. and six p. m. is of the greatest importance to the physician. It is also very essential that the frequency of the pulse be recorded at the same time the temperature is taken. The temperature of a typhoid patient, as a rule, rises on the average of one degree a day until it reaches 104 or 105 and even 106. However there are numerous deviations from the rule.

But the simple fact that there is no intermission of the fever and that the tendency is gradually upward, along with the other symptoms makes it easy to distinguish typhoid. As the fever rises there will be, as a rule, a corresponding increase in the frequency of the pulse of ten beats for each degree. However we have seen the pulse comparatively low while the temperature was high. About the beginning of the third week the pulse sometimes becomes rapid, rising to 130 or above, indicating weakness of the heart. So long as the pulse remains below 120 the outlook is favorable. The temperature, as a rule, rises steadily the first week, until it reaches its maximum, at which point it remains during the second week. If the case is doing well during the third week the temperature will be found decidedly lower in the morning and possibly an entire remission will be met. During the entire time of the fever the morning temperature will usually be one degree lower than the evening. A high morning temperature indicates a severe attack. A sudden fall of the temperature of several degrees in a few hours indicates internal hemorrhage. If this be true, there will be a blanching of the face and a rapid and great increase in the frequency of the pulse. As the temperature goes down the pulse goes up; just the reverse of the natural order which we have already mentioned. Hemorrhages usually occur during the second or third week.

In the course of the disease an ulceration takes place at several points in that part of the intestines already described. In the process of the ulceration blood vessels are eroded or eaten off and hemorrhages follow. If the blood vessels thus affected are small the hemorrhage will be slight, consisting of a mere oozing. If a large artery should be opened the hemorrhage may be so great as to affect the temperature and pulse, as described above, and even result in death.

Cold sweat on the forehead will also strongly confirm the suspicions of hemorrhage. A patient may die of internal hemorrhage without any blood appearing externally. In case symptoms of a pronounced hemorrhage occur the foot of the bed should be immediately elevated. A chair will generally answer the immediate necessity of keeping it elevated. A heavy towel rung out of the coldest water should be applied to the abdomen. If at hand an ice bag is better. Nothing hot or stimulating should be given. The readiest domestic remedy generally at hand is camphor. Put a few drops into a tablespoonful of water and give the patient. If reaction does not follow within ten minutes repeat the dose. Pond's extract or hamamelis is another domestic remedy usually at hand, of which teaspoonful doses may be given every fifteen minutes until the physician arrives.

The ulceration may be so great as to make an opening entirely through the wall of the intestine and allow its contents to escape into the abdominal cavity. This complication is called **perforation**. Perforation may occur any time during or after the third week and is indicated by a sudden attack of pain beginning just above the right groin and rapidly extending all over the abdomen. There is also a sudden seizure of diarrhœa and rapid distension of the abdomen. The case is then hopeless and death usually occurs within a few hours.

It is not unusual for the abdomen to be much distended during the regular course of an attack of typhoid, and so long as this condition remains, no matter how normal other conditions may be, the patient is not out of danger. When the fever is high, the abdomen hot and distended, a heavy towel wrung out of the coldest water and laid on will be beneficial. The towel may be reapplied as often as it gets warm.

Nose bleed occurs more frequently in typhoid than in any other disease.

Bronchitis frequently appears during the course of typhoid.

Treatment.—In no other disease is good nursing so essential. During the stage of delirium the patient must have the most faithful watching. During the latter stages the nurse must be ready for the emergencies occasioned by hemorrhages, as we have already described. At all times the nurse must religiously carry out thorough disinfection in the manner we have described. But it is in the feeding that the nurse must display the greatest firmness and show her loyalty to the physician. A little yielding on the part of the nurse to the patient's entreaties for food and the gratuitous but injurious advice of sympathetic friends, have cost many a life.

Diet.—All concede that the diet is the most essential part of the treatment in typhoid. But there is some difference of opinion as to what the diet should be.

Nine physicians out of ten give milk exclusively and, as a rule, force the patient to take the largest quantity possible. We obtain the most satisfactory results by giving absolutely no food whatever during the first week or until the temperature falls to 99 in the morning. Water is given freely. After the third day the hunger is not great. Whenever we are able to carry out this plan to the letter we find that the mind soon clears, the temperature sinks, the diarrhœa ceases, the abdomen becomes less sore and less distended. The tongue loses its irritable appearance, cleans and becomes moist and of a normal appearance. None of the more violent symptoms develop. No hemorrhage, no perforation and rarely a relapse. The symptoms all become so mild that the friends frequently doubt its being a genuine case of typhoid, or say, if it is typhoid, it is only a mild form of the disease.

We begin to feed by giving on the first day, every four hours, one tablespoonful of milk to which there has been added lime-water. The next day two tablespoonsful are given every four hours; the next three; the next four, and so on increasing until a large quantity is taken. Where milk is not borne well oat meal gruel may be given for a few days. The gruel should be prepared by cooking four hours and straining. Mutton broth is the first animal food allowed. No solid food is allowed until the temperature is normal in the evening for one week. Over feeding or a too early return to solid food is the most common cause of relapse.

Internal Remedies.—The homeopathic treatment is usually very satisfactory. Especially is this likely to be the case if the directions which we have given regarding diet are religiously observed. The remedies commonly indicated during a course of typhoid are Arsenicum, Baptisia, Belladonna, Bryonia, Gelsemium, Hyoscyamus, Phosphorus and Rhus Tox. Special symptoms may call for other remedies. When they are indicated can be determined by a careful study of the Materia Medica, Part II.

Belladonna.—The violent delirium always suggests this remedy. Any brain symptoms in the first stages of the disease is likely to demand it. Later in the disease it is not so useful.

Baptisia.—Most useful remedy. More frequently given in

the beginning than any other remedy. Brain symptom, prominent. Excessive drowsiness. Delirium. Confusion of ideas. Stupifying headache. Restless sleep. Head feels scattered about. Frightful dreams. Great debility. Answers slowly. Falls asleep while answering. Sensation as if in pieces. Sordes on teeth. Stool involuntary. Nose bleed. Besotted appearance. Chilly all day. Whole body feels sore. Imagines he can't get the pieces of his body together. Disposition to half close eyes. Can swallow liquids only; least solid food gags. Face flushed and dusky. Deaf. Disinclined to mental or bodily exertion. Sweat, urine and stool are extremely fetid.

Gelsemium.—At beginning of typhoid, when there are severe pains in the head, back and limbs. Great languor. Gets very tired between 4 and 5 p. m. Chilliness. Nervous chills, with chattering of teeth. Goose pimples. Typhoid in children. Nervous spasmodic movements. Twitching of the eyes. Fever without thirst. Trembling through whole body. Muscular prostration. Pain in neck and under left shoulder blade. Useful in first stage.

Bryonia.—While delirious continually talks about his business. Tries to get out of bed and says he wants to go home. Lips dry, brownish and cracked. Mouth very dry. Saliva frothy and soapy like. Great thirst. Faintness and nausea on sitting up. Kicks off the covers. Worse from motion. Constipated.

Hyoscyamus.—Delirium in the latter stages. Jumps out of bed and attempts to run away. Does not recognize relatives or friends. Sees persons who are not and have not been present. Delirious while awake. Constant staring. Very talkative. Eyes roll and squint. Urine and stool passed involuntarily. Sleepless. Jerking of tendons of wrist. Grating of teeth. Picking at bed clothes

Talks nonsense continually with eyes open. Pays no attention to any one. Starts up from sleep in a fright. Long continued sleeplessness, or constant sleep with muttering. Loss of speech. Tongue dry, red and cracked.

Phosphorus.—Bronchitis prominent. Brain exhaustion great. Sleeps continually. Typhoid pneumonia. Dry, annoying cough.

Rhus Tox.—Delirium mild. Bowels loose. Constantly tosses about; first on one side and then on the other. One moment lying down, another sitting up. Tongue has a triangular red tip. Stool passes during sleep; also urine. Dreams of something that requires muscular exertion on his part, as running. Pains in limbs worse when at rest. Dreams the moment he falls asleep. Answers slowly, but correctly.

Arsenicum.—Must not be given unless clearly indicated, as it will aggravate. Face pale, pinched and deathly. Lips dry, parched and black. Drinks little and often. Great anguish. Clammy forehead. Pulse rapid and feeble. Constantly licks the lips. Extremely weak. Foul odor from body. Slides down in bed and lower jaw drops down from weakness. Eyes sunken. Hot, red spot on cheek. Oppression of chest. Stool watery and foul. Skin dry, like parchment, or cold and moist. Usually indicated in latter stages of protracted cases.

TYPHUS FEVER.

This fever and typhoid were once supposed to be one and the same disease. The onset of typhus fever is sudden, the opposite of typhoid. It terminates abruptly within about two weeks, while typhoid subsides gradually after a course of three or more weeks.

It has a pronounced eruption, while typhoid has but little. Typhus is highly contagious, while typhoid is but slightly so. Nurses, doctors and all attendants upon a case of typhus usually take the disease. Typhus occurs where there are a large number of persons crowded together. Jail fever, ship fever and camp fever are a few of the many names under which typhus has been known. Overcrowding, lack of cleanliness, intemperance and lack of food are the predisposing causes. It rarely occurs in the United States. Occasional epidemics occur in the sea port cities. The usual source being a crowded emigrant vessel, although in 1877 typhus broke out in Montreal in the House of Refuge, which was so crowded in the basement that there were but eighty-eight cubic feet of air for each person; only five per cent. of the amount required to maintain good health. Typhus occurs frequently in Mexico, where the poverty and poor food favor its development. It is said to occur also in the rural districts as well as in the cities. This is explained by the fact that the natives inhabit small, damp and badly ventilated huts. It is supposed that the scourge which destroyed 800,000 Indians in Mexico in the year 1546 and increased the number to 2,000,000 in 1576, was no other than typhus.

Symptoms.—Onset sudden, about twelve days after exposure, chill or chills, recurring during first few days. Headache and pains in back and legs. Early prostration. Patient soon goes to bed. The temperature is high from the first; may reach the maximum, 104 to 106, the second day. Pulse, rapid. Tongue, parched and dry. Face, flushed. Eyes, congested. Expression, dull or stupid. Dizzy. Neuralgia above the eyes; lasts until second week. Nausea and vomiting. The latter may be distressing. There may be delirium. Skin dry and burning hot. Ringing in ears and deafness. Bowels constipated; diarrhœa, the exception. Urine diminished in quantity.

While the symptoms are all pronounced yet it is not until the eruption appears on the fifth day that the character of the disease can be determined. Eruption first appears upon the abdomen and upper part of chest, and then the face and extremities, developing so rapidly that in two or three days it is all out. The eruption has been described as having three parts; rose colored spots which disappear on pressure; dark red spots which are modified by pressure, and very tiny spots which are not affected by pressure. During the second week the symptoms are greatly aggravated and resemble very closely those occurring during the second or third week of a very severe case of typhoid. Typhus is sometimes mistaken for measles. Bronchitis is a frequent complication. Death occurs from blood poisoning and exhaustion toward end of second week. The mortality rate under old school treatment is from 20 to 50 per cent.

Treatment.—Study the remedies described for typhoid and the Materia Medica in Part II.

YELLOW FEVER.

This is an infectious and highly contagious disease, which derives its name from the jaundiced appearance of the skin usually seen during an attack of the disease. Cuba has been called its home, but it visits other regions which may be divided into three classes. Those from which it is never absent, including Havana, Vera Cruz, Rio and other Spanish-American ports. Those in which it recurs periodically, including the tropical Atlantic ports of America and Africa. Those in which it appears occasionally by accident, including the territory between latitudes 45 North and 35 South. The southern portion of the United States belongs to the last class. A strange fact is that while it has visited points upon or near the Atlantic coast, it has never visited the Pacific coast of America or Asia.

It rarely prevails in a region where the altitude is one thousand teet. It occurs only during the summer and autumn months in the United States. It is more prevalent in cities and more so in the poorer and unsanitary districts. It affects the natives less than foreigners. The mortality among negroes is much less than among whites. The mortality among whites ranges from 15 to 50 per cent. under old school treatment. During the epidemic of 1878 the reports from thirty cities showed a death rate everywhere among the whites between 40 and 50 per cent. The death rate of some 4000 cases treated homeopathically was less than 7 per cent. During the epidemic of 1888 the death rate under homeopathic treatment was less than 3 per cent. Having had the disease or having resided a long time where it prevails year after year, fortifies one against it. There are three forms, the mild, common and severe. There are three stages; the primary, the secondary and that of convalescence.

Symptoms.—May appear within one day after exposure to the infection, or may not until seven days. Average time, three or four days. Onset sudden and usually without any warning. A chill, commonly associated with pains in head, back and limbs. Throat sore. Nausea and vomiting; growing worse on second and third day. Fever rises rapidly. Skin dry and hot. Face hot. Tongue furred, but moist. Fever may be out of proportion to the other symptoms. Skin may be cool. Thirst, extreme. The pains in the back remind one of small-pox; but unlike small-pox, the eyes are red and watery. Bowels usually constipated. Delirium, in severe cases. Urine reduced and may be albuminous from the outset. After two or three days the fever subsides with all the other symptoms, and convalescence seems to be taking place. But it is only the beginning of the secondary stage or stage of calm. During this remission, or soon afterwards, the skin and eyes become quite yellow. In the mild form of the disease the patient will actually convalesce from this stage. But in the common form the temperature will rise again, beginning the third stage, during which the vomiting will be increased. In many cases the vomit will be of the color of tar, owing to the mixture of blood and the acid juices of the stomach. This is called the black vomit. The blood comes from the hemorrhages that take place from the walls of the stomach and intestines. The black vomit is not necessarily a fatal symptom, but it is present only in severe cases. Bleeding may occur from the kidneys, gums and under the skin.

In the severe form of the disease the patient usually dies within two or three days. Abscesses in various parts and diarrhœa may retard convalescence.

Treatment.—The patient should be placed in a well ventilated room and not allowed to sit up. The patient should not be kept in a state of perspiration.

While it may exhibit a commendable spirit for Northern nurses to volunteer to go South to nurse during an epidemic of yellow fever, it is not advisable, because they are not acclimated and are therefore most likely to be among the first victims.

In the medical treatment of this disease, as in all other diseases, the old school has been constantly changing. The most popular treatment with them at present is what is called the antacid or alkali plan. It consists in giving bi-carbonate of soda, mixed with some germicide like bichloride of mercury. The reason for the alkaline treatment is based on the fact that in this disease the contents of the stomach and intestines, the urine and the sweat are strongly acid. They have reached the conclusion to which the homeopaths arrived half a century ago, that quinine, opiates and stimulants are not only useless, but positively injurious. The vomiting may be lessened or controlled by cracked ice in the mouth and cold applications over the stomach.

Diet.—It is universally agreed that a yellow fever patient does best if no food whatever is given during the first stage. This coincides with our views in regard to feeding typhoid patients. While the stomach is in such an irritable state the presence of food would only aggravate.

Homeopathic Remedies.—For one who has carefully read the symptoms of the disease, and who has become thoroughly familiar with the Homeopathic Materia found in Part II, it would be easy to select the remedies most likely to be indicated in yellow fever. During the first stage Aconite, Belladonna, Bryonia or Gelsemium is likely to be needed. In the second stage the indications for Arsenicum or Lachesis are plain.

CEREBRO SPINAL FEVER.—(Meningitis.)

This is a specific, infectious disease, occurring here and there in epidemics. It is sometimes called spotted fever, also cerebro spinal meningitis. During the past three hundred years it has caused a great many deaths in Europe and America. It consists of an inflammation of the membranes covering the brain and spinal cord. It is more common among children than adults. Unhygienic surroundings favor its development; also over exertion, excessive heat, mental and bodily fatigue. The disease runs no regular definite course as typhoid and many other diseases, but appears under a variety of symptoms. It has been called a chameleon-like disease. Occurs more frequently in the winter and spring. Over-crowding favors its development. In this respect it is like typhus. The disease is supposed to be caused by a germ that is identical with those found in pneumonia. The mortality under old school treatment ranges from 30 to 75 per cent.

Symptoms.—The disease begins suddenly with a chill, nausea and vomiting. There is intense pain in the head, which soon extends to the back of the neck and down the spine, which is so agonizing that it soon renders the patient delirious. The pain in no other disease is so easily aggravated by light, noise and touch.

The very presence of another person annoys the patient. A seemingly peculiar fact is that notwithstanding the severe pain along the spine there is no tenderness in that region; even severe pressure is born without flinching, while slight pressure upon the stomach and other parts is usually painful. The skin is sensitive everywhere to a slight touch. The weight of the bed clothes is sufficient to cause pain. The delirium varies much in different cases. Often begins in a few hours. Several hours may elapse before the friends discover that the patient is not in his right mind. He may at first only display a difficulty in collecting his ideas and in answering questions. Later he becomes, as it were, sullen and morose, answering no questions. The delirium may be active from the beginning. The patient shouts, sings and attempts to do violence to himself or others. In this form the patient is more quiet during the day and more boisterous during the night.

If there is no delirium the patient is despondent and fearful, or may become stupid and unconscious.

The condition of the muscles affords some idea of the progress of the disease. Violent contractions of the muscles of the neck and back may occur, drawing the head backward. Hands and feet may be drawn into unusual positions, and any effort to straighten them causes pain. Paralysis does not often occur. Nausea and vomiting are usually among the first symptoms. The fever is at no time marked. At the beginning the temperature may be even below normal. In many cases blood escapes into the skin, causing spots from the size of a pin-head to a quarter of a dollar. It is from this appearance of the disease that it gets the name spotted fever. The pulse may vary thirty or forty beats within an hour. Vomiting is especially excited by rising.

The disease usually runs its course within a week. Death may occur within the first twenty-four hours. There are a number of affections with which the disease may be confounded; tubercular meningitis, cerebral complications of pneumonia, some phases of typhoid and even small-pox.

Treatment.—The old school authorities frankly confess that their resources for the treatment of cerebro spinal fever is exceedingly limited. Opium is their chief reliance. The symptoms of the disease correspond closely to the characteristic indications of a number of the homeopathic remedies, which have been given with satisfactory results. Study the following remedies in the Materia Medica in Part II: Apis, Argentum Nitr, Arnica, Bryonia, Cannabis Ind., Cimicifuga, Gelsemium, Glonion, Opium, Veratrum Virdie.

Gelsemium and Cimicifuga have been found especially valuable. Protracted recoveries may call for Calcarea Carb, Silicea and Sulphur.

RELAPSING FEVER.

This is a specific, infectious disease which runs a course of about six days and then there is an intermission of about six days. Then there is another rise of the fever which continues another five or six days. There may be three or even four relapses. It is from its peculiar relapsing feature that it derives its name. It has been called the "seven-day fever," also "famine fever," so called because it has been a frequent accompainment of famine in Ireland. It is common in India where the conditions for its development are always present. The germ which produces it has been determined. The disease has been produced in human beings and in monkeys by inoculation.

Symptoms.—The onset of the disease is abrupt. There is a chill and intense pain in back and limbs. There may be nausea, vomiting and convulsions in the young. Temperature rises rapidly, may reach 104 at end of first day. Sweats, common. Jaundice is common. Swelling of the spleen can be detected. The pulse is very rapid, ranging from 110 to 130. Stomach disturbances may be severe. There is not so much prostration as there is in typhoid and typhus. Patient may return to his work between relapses. Rarely delirium, and only when the temperature is very high. The temperature drops from the highest point to normal within a few hours. Each relapse is milder than the paroxysm that preceded it. The death rate is about four per cent.

The high temperature, the moist skin, the rapid pulse and the mildness of the other symptoms distinguish the disease from other fevers.

Treatment.—The following remedies, the indications of which are found in Part II, may be useful: Argenticum Nitr., Arsenicum, Bryonia, China, Eupatorium perf., Nux Vomica. The remedies mentioned under typhoid and intermittent fever should be studied and compared with the symptoms exhibited by the patient.

MALARIAL FEVER.

In the past the term malaria, like biliousness, has been a convenient one to apply to a number of obscure troubles that puzzled the physician to diagnose. However, the bright light of scientific research has found that malarial fever is a definite disease due to a specific parasite which inhabits the blood corpuscles and is therefore named hæmatozoa, meaning a blood animal. Whether one has or has not malaria can be definitely determined by a microscopic examination of the blood. Even approaching paroxysms of the disease can be predicted from the microscopic appearances of the parasites in freshly drawn blood from the patient.

Malaria may manifest itself in four distinct forms: Intermittent fever, continued remittent fever, pernicious malarial fever and chronic malarial poisoning.

Intermittent Fever.—This form is distinguished by recurring paroxysms, consisting of a chill, fever and sweat in succession. The patient is usually warned of the approaching chill by unpleasant and uneasy feelings, consisting of a feeling of lassitude, a desire to stretch and yawn, headache and sometimes nausea and vomiting. Even before the chill the thermometer will show a slight rise in the temperature. Gradually the patient begins to shiver and perhaps the teeth will chatter and the whole body shakes so as to move the bed. The patient looks cold and blue. The skin will be cold, but the thermometer will show the temperature several degrees above normal, 105 or 106. The chill lasts from ten minutes to an hour. Headache may be intense. The chill completes the cold stage. The hot stage immediately follows. First, flushes of heat, gradually warming up of the surface until it becomes burning hot. The pulse, which was small and rapid, now becomes full and bounding. The heart beats with great force, and there may be a severe, throbbing headache. But the real temperature shown by the thermometer may not be any greater than it was during the chill. The hot stage continues from a half hour to three or four hours. The thirst for cold water is usually very great during the hot stage, and but little during the cold stage. However there are cases where the reverse of this occurs. The careful homeopathic prescriber will always endeavor to ascertain during which stage the thirst is present. The sweating stage follows the hot stage and is indicated by a profuse sweat. Usually within an hour or two all the disagreeable symptoms of the preceding stages disappear and the patient drops off into a refreshing sleep, completing a paroxysm. The periodical return of these paroxysms within twelve, twenty-four, forty-eight or seventy-two hours, is a striking characteristic of this form of malarial fever. The paroxysms usually recur every day or every other day. The disease may run a course of ten days or two weeks and disappear of its own accord, but it may persist indefinitely, in which case the blood becomes very poor and the skin jaundiced. It may run on into chronic malarial poisoning, which we have already mentioned as the fourth form of malaria.

We will describe it after disposing of the second and third forms. In different countries intermittent fever is known by several popular names. "Fever and ague," "chills and fever," "swamp fever," "shakes," "Panama fever." The symptoms and severity varies in different countries, but the essential features are always the same. It occurs more frequently in low, swampy districts, yet, in some of the greatest swamps, it has been unknown. It is rapidly disappearing from the Northern states. This disappearance seems to be coincident with the clearing-up and settling of the country.

Continued Remittent form of malarial fever has no distinct intermission of the fever, but has a decided remission during which the temperature drops nearly to the normal, but never completely. This form of malarial fever is also known by the names bilious remittent fever, remittent fever, bilious remittent and typho-malarial fever. This form of malarial fever may set in with a definite chill or may be preceded a few days by a feeling of lassitude. On the second or third day the patient has a flushed face, and a temperature of 102 or 103. The tongue is furred and the pulse full and bounding. There will be many other symptoms suggesting typhoid fever. There is often slight bronchitis.

The fever continues with more or less marked remissions. Definite paroxysms with or without chill may occur. The temperature may reach 105 or 106. The intestinal symptoms common to typhoid are absent. There may be jaundice. Delirium, if present, will be slight. The fever may subside completely at the end of a week or may continue two weeks. It is often difficult to distinguish it from typhoid. From this fact it has sometimes been called typho-malarial fever. In some cases the remissions become so slight and the fever so continuous that physicians of large experience will scarcely be able to distinguish it from typhoid. The absence of the bowel symptoms peculiar to typhoid will be the chief distinguishing point.

An absolute diagnosis can be made by microscopical examination of the blood by an expert who is familiar with the parasite causing malaria. While it is well to know this fact it is not often practical to secure such an examination.

Pernicious Malarial Fever.—This form of malaria is rare in the temperate climates. It is believed by some to be only a more severe form of remittent fever. There are three types: The comatose, the algid and the hemorrhagic. The first begins with violent brain disturbance, which is soon followed by a rapidly developing stupor. The unconsciousness may last six, twelve or twenty-four hours. The patient may die during the attack or may become unconscious and suffer from a second paroxysm, proving fatal. The *algid* type is characterized by great disturbances of the stomach and coldness. There may be no actual chill, but the prostration is very great. The temperature may be normal or below normal. Pulse, feeble. Respirations, rapid. Mind usually clear. Urine scanty or suppressed. Patient dies within a few days of exhaustion. The *hemorrhagic* type is characterized by a bleeding from the mucous membrane. Other types occur.

Pernicious malarial fever has been known as African fever, Jungle fever, Hungarian fever, and in the South during the war it was known as Chickahominy fever.

Chronic Malarial Poisoning.—The symptoms of this form of malaria are varied. It frequently follows the remittent form of malaria, where it has been badly or imperfectly treated. After several attacks of the intermittent form the patient's blood becomes so impoverished by the destructive ravages of the parasites that we have the condition known as the chronic form of malaria, consisting of breathlessness on exertion, swelling of the ankles, hemorrhages, especially in the eye, saffron colored skin, and enlarged spleen.

Chronic malarial poisoning is also indicated by the regular return of neuralgia in some part every day or every other day. The fact that any symptom or complaint is worse at *regular* times suggests malaria. Absence of feeling in certain parts, itching, burning, tingling or numbness may be symptoms of the same trouble. Symptoms which make the patient think of paralysis are often due to malaria. A chronic morning diarrhœa may have a malarial origin. So may catarrh and hemorrhages from various parts be due to the same cause.

Treatment.—Recovery from malarial fever and the disappearance of the parasites from the blood are coincident, no matter whether the recovery be spontaneous or the result of the action of drugs. It would seem then that the rational treatment of malaria would be that which would destroy the germs or cause them to disappear. The most certain way to destroy or cause to emigrate anything that has life, whether it be colonies of parasites or colonies of human beings, is to deprive them of their natural nutrition; in other words render sterile or non-productive the soil upon which they live. Experiments have been made showing that quinine, in a solution of 1 to 20,000, will destroy parasites similar to those of malaria within two hours, the effect upon them being manifest within five minutes. It has also been shown that quinine affects greatly the material from which the parasites develop and upon which they feed. Five grains of quinine equally distributed in the entire quantity of blood of an adult would make a dilution of the proportion of 1 to 16,000.

It is said that when quinine is taken into the body it at once enters into the blood vessels and circulates with the blood. It is also said that the active parasites of malaria are found only within the blood vessels, just as the germs of diphtheria are found, only in the throat. Such are the results reached by the latest scientific researches in the domain of medicine. But quinine for "chills and fever" has been used for a long time, in fact, it is the one universal remedy for malaria used by all, excepting the homeopaths. Our old school friends frequently speak of quinine curing malaria as being the one thing in medicine of which they were absolutely positive.

Peruvian bark, from which quinine is made, was unknown previous to the middle of the seventeenth century. The Jesuits in Peru distributed it among the poor as a remedy for fever. It was in the year 1790, while investigating the properties of the drug, that Hahnemann observed that it produced in persons in perfect health symptoms similar to those for which it had been given. It was then that the homeopathic law of cure dawned upon his mind, and he began to investigate other drugs and note their effects upon well persons. He soon discovered that the Peruvian or quinine bark was only curative in malaria having certain symptoms. For instance: Chill, preceded by thirst, but no thirst during hot stage following. Thirst again during the sweating stage. These and many other symptoms found in the Materia Medica, Part II, determine in what cases of malarial fever China, a homeopathic remedy derived from the Peruvian bark, is indicated and in what cases it will not prove beneficial.

A close study of the Homeopathic Materia Medica reveals the fact that there are a score or more of remedies as useful in malarial fever as China; in fact, several are more frequently indicated. The question arises: Does quinine really cure malaria? Is it not a palliative? The difference between the curative and palliative action of a drug is discussed under the General Remarks in the beginning of this volume. Quinine poisoning is known to be of frequent occurrence. It has been known to seriously impair the hearing and affect other organs injuriously. It is a fact that many cases occur in which the heaviest doses of quinine seem to make no impression upon the chills and fever. We have seen cases that have been taking quinine for years. Is it not possible that the quinine simply suppresses the disease for the time being? In many cases, just as soon as the quinine is abandoned, the chills and fever return. This would indicate that the drug is only palliative and not curative. And in some cases it is not even palliative. This is the conclusion reached by every thorough homeopath. The universal habit of taking quinine not only for malaria, but for almost every other complaint, is a pernicious one. It must necessarily do a vast amount of harm. It undoubtedly suppresses or perverts many of the functions of the body. We know that the quinine habit is the unsuspected source of a large number of troubles. The poor sufferer complains and complains, but he keeps on taking his quinine year in and year out.

The abundant resources of homeopathy for curing malaria stand out in striking contrast with the one palliative resource of the old school.

No other class of diseases will test one's practical knowledge of homeopathy so thoroughly, and in no other disease will the correct homeopathic prescription be followed by such marvelous results. We have seen cases of chronic malaria of a dozen years standing cured by a few doses of Sulphur, or a few doses of Natrum Mur.; cases which had been taking quinine continually for years.

In chronic malarial troubles of long standing, especially where much quinine has been taken, **Natrum Mur.** is very frequently indicated. There is thirst with chill or cold spell every day or every other day between 10 and 11 a. m. The coldness is first felt in the feet and finger tips. The lips and nails turn blue. The cold stage is followed by heat and bursting headache. In the cases needing this remedy there is usually a great craving for salt. An extra amount of salt must be put into the food. It will be remembered that this remedy is the common table salt homeopathically prepared. In it we have an illustration of the fact that a substance in its crude form may have no medicinal powers, but when highly diluted may develop some of the most remarkable remedial qualities. **Sulphur** is called for in these troubles when there is faint spell every day between 10 and 11 a. m. The top of the head is hot and aches. There are flushes and the feet are so hot that they must be uncovered at night when in bed.

The following are a few of the more frequently indicated homeopathic remedies for malarial fever: Apis, Arnica, Arsenicum, Belladonna, Bryonia, China, Eupatorium perf., Gelsemium, Ignatia (thirst only during chill), Natrum Mur., Podophyllum, Pulsatilla, Rhus Tox, Sulphur and Veratrum Virdie. For particular indications for each remedy, see Materia Medica in Part II.

DENGUE FEVER.

This is an acute infectious disease which was first noticed in Java about a hundred years ago. It first appeared in America after the landing of a cargo of slaves from Africa. It has been called African fever, also break-bone or dandy fever. It is confined to the tropical and subtropical regions. Epidemics have recently prevailed in Egypt and Texas. Many regard it as highly contagious. It is conveyed by ships and along railroads. It usually attacks every member in the community in which it appears, excepting those who have previously had the disease. The particular germ that produces it has not yet been determined. Some think that the disease is a mild form of yellow fever, while others would class it with malarial.

Symptoms.—The attack sets in gradually, with headache, watering of eyes, chilly feelings and intense aching pain in the joints and muscles. The most distressing symptom is the breakbone pains, which is more agonizing than in any other disease. Even more severe than those of small-pox and yellow fever. The neuralgia or rheumatism element is the most prominent feature of the disease. The fever rises gradually and may reach 106 or higher on the third or fourth day. It then gradually subsides during the next two or three days, after which there is all the appearance of convalesence, only to be followed within a few days by another paroxysm perhaps more severe than the first. In its remission it reminds one of relapsing fever. Between the two paroxysms, about the fifth or sixth day from the beginning, an eruption breaks out, often resembling measles, but of no uniform character. It is peculiar in that it first appears upon the palms of the hand, then upon the neck and then extends downward over the rest of the body. The eruption may at times resemble that of scarlet fever. The swelling of the glands is a feature quite peculiar to dengue and distinguishes it from many other diseases with which it might be confounded. First those in the groin swell and then those under the arm and about the neck. They enlarge rapidly and become very tender. They remain swollen until all the other symptoms subside. The stiffness of the joints and the prostration that follows the disappearance of the more violent symptoms are very marked.

Treatment.—While the disease is rarely if ever fatal, it requires treatment. In the beginning, **Aconite**; if brain symptoms are prominent, **Belladonna**; for the vomiting, **Ipecac**; for the wandering pains, **Pulsatilla**; for the fixed local pains, **Rhus Tox**; and during convalescence, **China**.

INFLUENZA (La Grippe).

The grip, as popularly called, is an infectious disease, in which catarrh of the mucous membranes is usually a prominent symptom. The disease has been known for several centuries under different names. Several epidemics have occurred which have swept over the whole civilized world within a remarkably short period. Within a few weeks it has spread over an entire continent. Epidemics occurred in 1833, 1847-48, 1889-90 and also 1890-91. Many of the epidemics have started in Russia, from which fact it has sometimes been called the Russian fever. In October, 1889, it appeared in St. Petersburg and two months later it was epidemic in America. This reminds us that the cholera epidemic of '92 proceeded in a similar manner. The real cause of the disease is as yet undetermined. A germ resembling that of pneumonia has been frequently found in grip cases.

Symptoms.—Resembles those of any ordinary cold in which there is fever, dryness and stuffiness of the nose, along with considerable catarrh of the throat and lungs. There is usually at the outset severe headache and pain in the back and limbs, along with general soreness. This feature reminds one of small-pox and dengue fever. Delirium may be great. A common characteristic of the disease is to manifest itself at the weakest point. Whether it be the heart, the lungs, the kidneys, or some other organ. Latent weaknesses are invariably aggravated and for this reason, sooner or later, fatal results often follow the disease. Pneumonia is one of its most frequent and fatal complications. Abscesses of the brain and of the lung have followed it; also, mental derangement. Fatal Bright's disease has suddenly developed as one of its direct after effects. Weak hearts have frequently and suddenly given out under its influence. Catarrh of the stomach and intestines, causing diarrhœa, are often prominent symptoms.

Treatment.—As a rule, a person in whom every organ is sound, has little to fear from this disease, but those in whom there is any weakness may be affected seriously. Every case should be treated as a serious one. The patient should be put to bed and kept there until the fever has completely disappeared. Going out too soon while convalescing from this disease is very likely to be followed by a relapse worse than the original attack. The person who tries to keep on at his work while having the grip makes a very great if not a fatal mistake.

Between the last epidemic and the one preceding it there was an interval of more than forty years. Therefore when the epidemic of 1889 and '90 appeared but few of the physicians in practice had ever seen a case of the grip. A remarkable opportunity to compare the merits of the old and new school treatment was presented. The allopaths had no invariable law to guide them. Their prescriptions were necessarily crude experiments and it is not strange, therefore, that the mortality under their treatment was enormous. On the other hand the advantage of the homeopaths having a universal and unvarying law by which to guide them was more apparent than ever. The homeopaths took hold of the disease as readily and were as successful in treating it as if they had always been familiar with it. They were as successful in the beginning of the epidemic as they were at its close. Their mortality was nothing compared with that of the old school. In Buffalo, N. Y., statistics show that the allopathic mortality rate was six times as great as the homeopathic. The cases that had homeopathic treatment exclusively were rarely complicated or followed by serious after effects. The secret of the homeopath's success was that he knew his Materia Medica and whatever symptoms were presented he found no difficulty in finding a remedy that was adapted to them. While the contrast between the two schools was strikingly presented in that epidemic it must not be forgotten that the same difference always exists. The universality and flexibility in its application of the homeopathic law enables the homeopathic prescriber to more readily adapt the remedy to the case, no matter what it may be, nor does it make any particular difference in the prescription whether or not he has ever seen another case like it. At the beginning of the last epidemic every homeopathic physician in general practice treated many cases successfully before he knew he was really treating the grip.

Remedies.—A significant fact is that after the epidemic was over when Drs. Smith, Jones, Brown and others came to compare notes, they found that notwithstanding their respective fields of practice were located thousands of miles apart, their treatment had been substantially the same. They had given **Bryonia** more often, perhaps, than any other remedy; because the symptoms of the disease more often corresponded to those found in the Materia Medica under Bryonia. They also found at times **Gelsemium, Eupatorium, Rhus Tox** or **Belladonna** indicated, and gave each when indicated, with equally good results.

We saw congestion of the brain, with high fever and delirium, speedily relieved by **Veratrum Virdie.**

Camphor taken at the beginning of the attack lightened and shortened it. **Nux Vomica** was also valuable as a preventive of the disease. In the next epidemic other symptoms may call for other remedies, which can readily be determined by a study of the Materia Medica, Part II.

MUMPS.

This is an infectious disease which manifests itself by an inflammation of the parotid gland, which is located just back of the angle of the jaw and in front of the lower half of the ear. The particular germ always present in this disease has been described. Mumps occurs as an epidemic; more prevalent in the spring and autumn. It is more common in children and youths. Very young children and adults usually escape it. More frequently met among males than females.

Symptoms.—The disease appears two or three weeks after exposure to the infection. There is a slight fever, about 101. The child complains of a pain just in front of the ear on one side. A slight swelling is noticed at that point, which gradually increases for forty-eight hours. At the end of which time the side of the neck and face are considerably swollen. The glands under the jaw may also become much swollen. Within a day or two the other side of the face and neck become involved. The patient finds it difficult to eat or talk. The swelling subsides in a week or ten days.

Occasionally the disease is severe. In which case there may be high fever, delirium and great prostration. Within a few weeks we have had three such cases under our care. Each case seemed to be a relapse, from exposure during convalescence, from the first attack. But instead of the parotid gland the testicle was the seat of pain and swelling. The suffering was great. In females it occasionally affects the breasts and ovaries.

Treatment.—The diet must necessarily be liquid. The lighter and less stimulating it is the better. The patient should remain quiet within doors and free from exposure. In case of great swelling of the testicle with severe pain we have seen prompt relief from the following evaporating lotion: Mix two drachms of the Muriate of Amonia, two ounces of alcohol and two ounces of water; apply by saturating a thin piece of gauze and loosely wrapping it about the part. The chief internal remedy is **Mercurius.** Its tendency to act upon the glands is well known. **Aconite, Belladonna** and **Pulsatilla** may be needed. The iodide of mercurius is probably the best form in which to use the drug. We saw the most happy result follow a few doses of **Belladonna** in a case where there was delirium and a scarlet red face. **Pulsatilla** is likely to be needed in case of complications in females.

WHOOPING COUGH.

The name of this disease indicates the character of its cough. The "whoop" is produced during a prolonged drawing in of the breath. A germ has been found with the disease which, when cultivated and inoculated into animals, produces a catarrhal condition not unlike that which accompanies the disease in the human subject. Whooping cough usually prevails in the winter and spring, often preceding or following an epidemic of measles. It occurs more frequently among children between six months and six years. Girls are more liable to have it than boys. In this respect it is the opposite of mumps. Young infants and the aged may have the disease and result fatally. The death rate among negroes is twice as great as it is among the whites. It will be remembered that in yellow fever the reverse is true.

Symptoms.—The attack comes on within a week or ten days after exposure. At first the patient seems to have only an ordinary cold. There is slight fever, the nose runs and the eyes are red. There is usually a dry, spasmodic cough. After a week or ten days more the peculiar "whoop" is heard. The fit of coughing begins with a number of short coughs in rapid succession, leading up to the "whoop." A little stringy mucus is discharged as a result of the coughing or vomiting. There may be but a few fits of coughing a day or in severe cases there may be several. During a fit of coughing the face gets blue, the eyes stand out and suffocation threatens. But at this juncture the air which was temporarily shut off enters the lungs with a deep crowing sound called the "whoop." Children soon learn to dread the fit or paroxysm of coughing and endeavor to escape from it when they feel that one is coming on. After continuing three or four weeks the symptoms gradually subside. One attack prevents a second. It is much less contagious than measles. Rarely carried by clothing. Excessive vomiting and diarrhœa complicate the disease. Fatal hemorrhages have occured during the fits of coughing. Pneumonia is one of the worst complications. In England it ranks third among the fatal diseases of children. The general mortality rate is from 3 to 5 per cent. But the rate among children during the second year has reached as high as 48 per cent. Whooping cough is, therefore, a more serious disease than is commonly supposed, and should be carefully treated as such. At this point we are reminded of the death of a beautiful boy one year of age from whooping cough. Up to that time the parents, and the writer, too, had shared in the popular belief that it was a mild affection and underestimated its gravity. The disease in this case progressed with less attention than it would have received had it been something else. An uncontrollable vomiting and diarrhœa set in, the result of brain disturbances, and death soon followed.

Treatment.—There should be protection from cold and everything else likely to aggravate the trouble. The diet should be light and unstimulating. A vegetable diet is best. The less meat the better. Any food hard to digest should be avoided. The remedies required in the first stage are the same as would be indicated in any case of cold, catarrh and cough. The following will be frequently needed: *Aconite, Pulsatilla, Mercurius, Belladonna, Nux Vom., Ipecac.* **Belladonna** given persistently from the beginning of the attack until the end is all that is necessary in some cases. During the second stage the following may be indicated: *Arsenicum, Drosera, Tartar Emetic or Veratrum Alb.* During the third or convalescing stage after the whooping has disappeared and there remains only a dry, hacking cough, **Phosphorus** will be of service. Coldness, paleness, weakness, thirst and worse about midnight will suggest **Arsenicum**. Attacks of coughing in rapid succession, with warm perspiration on forehead, **Drosera**. Vomiting with every coughing spell, **Tartar Emetic**. Coughing and vomiting spells in which the child falls over from exhaustion and in which the forehead is covered with cold sweat along with diarrhœa, will indicate **Veratrum Alb.**

ASIATIC CHOLERA.

This most fatal disease is now known to be caused by a germ called the comma bacillus, discovered by Dr. Koch in 1884. Its most striking feature is the vomiting and purging. Volumes could be written upon its history. It has prevailed in India from a remote period, but not until the present century has it appeared in Europe and America. In 1817 36,000 persons in Calcutta were attacked with the disease within three months. An English army of 90,000 men, marching through India, lost 9000 within twelve days. For the next fifteen years from that date cholera proceeded, for the first time, westward, by a series of epidemics, until it had reached nearly every portion of the civilized world. It reached America for the first time in 1832 by Quebec, also by New York. There were recurrences in 1835 and '36. In 1841 another great epidemic broke out in India. It reached Europe in 1847, spreading through Russia first, and then Germany, England and France. America was reached in 1848 by way of New Orleans, spreading up the Mississippi Valley and across the continent to California.

It appeared again in 1849. A third great outbreak occurred in India in 1850, entering Europe in 1853. In 1854 it was introduced into New York by emigrant vessels and a severe epidemic spread extensively over North and South America. In 1865 the disease appeared in Arabia and Egypt, crossed to Constantinople in July and reached England in the autumn. The following year it appeared in America. In 1873 it again reached the United States, but did not prevail extensively. In 1884 there was another outbreak in Europe. During the summer of 1892 it prevailed extensively in Russia, causing, perhaps, 100,000 deaths. Later in the summer it was epidemic at Hamburg. A large number of cases occurred in France and a few cases reached England. There was also a number of deaths on board of emigrant vessels which arrived in New York. The rigid quarantine and the cold weather arrested it for the time being. Whether it will become epidemic or not the coming season, during the Columbian World's Fair year, is the question of the hour.

Cholera is not so highly contagious as measles or small-pox, but more like typhoid fever. Physicians, nurses and others in close contact with the patient do not, as a rule, take the disease. Impure drinking water is believed to be the chief source of the infection. In this respect it is similar to typhoid. Some maintain that certain conditions of the soil favor its development, especially when a very dry spell follows a very wet one. Hot weather favors its development. Yet most epidemics in America and Europe have occurred in late summer and autumn. It occurs less frequently in high altitudes. It attacks persons of all ages and particularly those who are intemperate and debilitated by lack of food and proper hygienic surroundings. One attack does not prevent a second.

Symptoms.—The disease manifests itself from two to five days after the infection has been received into the system. There are three stages. The preliminary diarrhœa, the collapse stage and the period of reaction. *The preliminary diarrhœa* is usually preceded for a few hours or for a few days by colicky pains, with a rumbling in the abdomen. Nausea, vomiting, looseness of the bowels and mental depression are not uncommon, but the preliminary diarrhœa or first stage may set in abruptly without any of these warnings. This diarrhœa is usually mild and painless, such as might come on after any little indiscretion in diet and is apt to be considered a matter of no importance. But it continues and in the morning or middle of the night the *second* stage is ushered in by a profuse diarrhœa in which the discharges pass away in a stream. After one or two evacuations the discharges lose their customary odor and color, becoming "rice water" like in appearance. There will be from three to twenty evacuations a day. With each evacuation there may be vomiting of matter resembling that evacuated from the bowels. As a rule the patient suffers none of the distress usually incident to vomiting or diarrhœa. Rapid exhaustion comes on, with an unquenchable thirst. The pulse is very rapid; the skin shrunken, cool or clammy, and the extremities blue. The complexion is ashy grey, the nose pinched, the cheeks hollow and the eyeballs sunken in their sockets. The temperature in the mouth will be from five to ten degrees below normal, while that of the rectum is 103 or 104. The temperature under the arm may fall to 72, while that of the rectum is above a hundred. The patient does not complain of feeling cold. The sweat makes the patient appear colder than he really is. Headache and dizziness are sometimes present. The tongue is white. There are severe cramps in the legs and feet which cause the patient to shriek. The breathing is irregular and of a sighing character. The patient gasps for breath. Air expelled from the mouth is cold. The voice becomes hoarse, or there is only a husky whisper. The mind is usually clear throughout, but the patient does not realize the gravity of his case. He has no fears. There is no saliva in the mouth and the urine is suppressed. Possibly a few albuminous drops may pass. Later the discharges may be less frequent and have the odor of decayed fish. This stage of collapse may last for forty-eight hours and yet the patient recover. If recovery does take place the third or *reactive stage* now sets in rapidly. The blueness gradually disappears. Warmth returns. The heart action becomes stronger and the pulse becomes perceptible. The urine increases. The irritability of the stomach subsides. The stools are less frequent. But relapse and death may occur during this stage. The condition known as *cholera typhoid* often occurs after several days of apparent convalescence. The patient becomes delirious and presents many other symptoms common to typhoid. A fatal poisoning may occur from a failure of the urine to secrete. Numerous other complications may occur. Death may occur within twelve hours from the beginning of the attack. Death may occur without any great evacuations from the bowels. Cholera need not be confounded with any other disease. A case of poisoning will have great distress from vomiting, while cholera has none. The stool in case of poisoning will be mucous and blood stained. Those of cholera are of a " rice water " character. In a case of cholera a microscopical examination of the discharges will reveal the presence of the specific germ of cholera.

The death rate in cholera, under old school treatment, ranges from 30 to 80 per cent. In the epidemic of 1832 in Germany the allopathic mortality rate was over 31 per cent.; the homeopathic rate under 7 per cent. In the epidemic of 1848, in Scotland, the allopathic death rate was 84 per cent., while that of the homeopaths was 24. In 1849, in Cincinnati, the homeopathic rate was less than 4 per cent., so low and so unusual that it was publicly questioned and investigated. The fact was verified. Last year, in

Hamburg, the homeopathic loss was less than 5 per cent., while the allopathic was over 42. Total average, allopathy, 51.3; homeopathy, 8.8.

Before Hahnemann ever saw a case of cholera he predicted correctly the remedies that would be found most useful in the disease. Any one who understands the homeopathic law and who is thoroughly familiar with the homeopathic Materia Medica can do the same in respect to any disease he has never seen or treated, provided he is given an accurate description of the symptoms that accompany it.

Treatment.—In cholera times all drinking water should be boiled before using; milk or any other liquid should be treated in the same way. All food should be cooked and care taken not to overeat. Excessive mental and physical exertion should be avoided, as well as stimulants and late hours. If any looseness of the bowels occur the patient should go to bed immediately and remain there quiet until over it. Diarrhœa of any kind is more quickly overcome by abstaining entirely from all food.

In no other disease is prompt action more important. Much can and must be done before the physician arrives. Every person attacked with colic, diarrhœa, vomiting or any other symptom suggestive of cholera, should at once take Camphor. Put one drop of the tincture upon a lump of sugar and repeat the dose every fifteen minutes until relief is certain. Very often no other remedy will be required. Camphor, given at the *beginning*, is invaluable. Later on in the disease it is useless. A bottle of homeopathic pills, medicated with camphor, should always be carried with one during the prevalence of cholera. The particular symptoms calling for camphor are as follows: Nose cold and pinched; cold sweat on face, with vomiting; tongue cold, flabby and trembling; terrible anguish and burning at pit of stomach driving to despair; anxiety and restlessness; feeling as if cold air were blowing on parts covered; eyes sunken and fixed; sudden sinking and loss of strength; icy coldness of the whole body; lips purple and drawn; pulse scarcely perceptible; cold extremities; very sensitive to cold air, skin becomes very cold; cold, clammy, weakening sweat; sighing respiration.

If Camphor fails to arrest the disease **Veratrum album** is the next remedy generally indicated. The special symptoms calling for it are: Cold sweat on forehead; diarrhœa frequent, profuse and gushing, with severe, pinching, colicky pains; rice water discharges; purging and vomiting simultaneously; frequent watery vomiting, especially after drinking; cramps in calves and fingers; constant desire for cold drinks and acids; violent colic and rumbling in abdomen; skin in palms wrinkled; great weakness after vomiting, faints; blue lips and great dark circles about the eyes.

Cuprum is indicated where the cramping is especially prominent. Cramps occur not only in the calves, feet, toes and fingers, but in the stomach and chest. The face is distorted and the voice is lost. There is difficulty in swallowing; the breathing, labored, and the urine, suppressed. When the skin is pinched up it remains in the same position, inelastic. Cuprum is the best preventive of cholera. When cholera is prevailing take half a dozen pellets of Cuprum 6x every other day. This remedy is prepared from copper. It is said that those who work in copper usually escape the disease. Copper plates have been worn over the abdomen as a preventive.

Arsenicum is indicated when the attack comes on suddenly with great prostration and restlessness. Great burning in the stomach, with intense thirst and vomiting as soon as drink is taken are strong indications for this remedy.

Carbo Veg is indicated when the cramps and discharges have ceased and the patient lies in a stupor, pulseless; a perfect picture of collapse; cold tongue, cold breath and cold all over. It is said to have saved many cases in the last stage, when death seemed inevitable. The 30 x is the best form in which to give it.

During convalescence symptoms for a number of remedies may occur. **Bryonia** and **Rhus Tox** are frequently indicated in the typhoid form. **China** is often of service during convalescence. It is always indicated after any great loss of vital fluids. It should be remembered that too much camphor can be given. During convalescence nearly as much care is needed in feeding as during recovery from typhoid. The same directions will hold good in both cases. Over feeding in either case may cost a life. Washing out the bowels several times with two or three quarts of warm **soap suds** has recently been strongly advocated. The measure commends itself to us as being at least a useful aid, since soap is one of the best **disinfectants**. It must not be forgotten that the same care in disinfecting the discharges and soiled linen in a cholera case is needed as in a case of typhoid. Here again the same directions will answer for both.

Ipecacuanha.—May be indicated in the milder cases where nausea and vomiting are the most prominent symptoms. The matter vomited and the stools are grass-green.

ERYSIPELAS.

Many erroneously regard as erysipelas any redness of the skin accompanied with heat. True erysipelas is an acute inflammation of the skin, caused by a germ which is identical with one of the germs that produces pus. The inflammation may occur on any part of the body, but is more frequently found on the face. The disease is more prevalent in the spring and more likely to occur in old buildings with unhygienic surroundings. It is contagious and may be communicated by a third person. It does not possess a high degree of contagiousness. One may be inoculated with it. The infection may cling to the walls, furniture, bedding and other articles of a room that has been occupied by an erysipelas patient. Persons with wounds of any kind are more likely to take the disease. Women who have recently been confined are very susceptible to the contagion. A physician should not take care of a confinement case and one of erysipelas at the same time. Many persons are accustomed to repeated attacks of the disease; recurring every year or two. A number of complications occur which may terminate fatally.

Symptoms.—The disease manifests itself from two to seven days after exposure or contact with the infection. There is usually a severe chill, followed by a rapid rise of temperature. At some point the skin will be slightly reddened. This will increase and within twenty-four hours the skin will be red, shiny and swollen. The inflamed skin will be clearly marked off by a difference of color from that which is not. The outer layer of the skin is often raised in blisters containing water or matter. If the disease is located on the face the swelling will begin on one side and extend to the other, perhaps, closing both eyes during its course. Even in mild cases, the face, including eye-lids and ears, is enormously swollen and so distorted that the patient is scarcely recognizable. The parts first affected gradually become pale, while other parts are becoming inflamed. The fever remains high without intermission for four or five days. The disease may extend to distant parts. Various complications may occur. In severe cases there may be delirium. But the presence of delirium does not always indicate brain complications. Persons who are otherwise in good health rarely die from the disease.

Treatment.—The patient should be isolated. Many cases will recover without any treatment. The diet should be light and unstimulating. No meat should be allowed. Here, again, the homeopathic treatment is infinitely superior to that of the old school. **Belladonna** is especially indicated in erysipelas of the face when the color is a bright red. Other symptoms indicating this remedy are: A throbbing headache; delirium; congestion to the head; skin smooth, red and shining; redness begins in small spots and extends in streaks; light and noise unbearable; worse at 3 p. m. **Arsenicum** is indicated when the skin has a blackish hue, along with this condition there is: Great prostration; great thirst; great restlessness; burning pains; worse about midnight. **Rhus Tox** is also frequently needed for the little watery blisters and the intolerable burning, itching and tingling. We have seen persons who were subject to repeated attacks, cured by **Sulphur.** Not only cured, but the duration of the attack was only one-fourth of the usual time. Other remedies are often indicated. We recall a case where there was delirium and incessant talking. A single prescription of **Stramonium** 200 speedily cured it.

BLOOD POISONING.

The scientific names expressing the conditions known commonly as blood poisoning, are Septicæmia and Pyæmia. Blood poisoning is due to the absorption of poisonous material produced by bacteria. The particular germs are known as streptococci and staphylococci. Within a few hours after a wound there often occurs a fever, rising rapidly to 103 or 104, but quickly subsiding. It is not preceded by a chill and no serious constitutional disturbances take place. It is supposed to be caused by the absorption of certain ferments from the blood. But when the products of the putrefactive germs are absorbed through the wound, a chill occurs twenty-four or forty-eight hours after the accident or operation. The fever rapidly rises to 103 or 104. The pulse is quick. Headache, restlessness and delirium are common. The tongue is dry and glazed. The symptoms vary according to the amount of poison absorbed.

When the germ, as well as their poisonous products, enter the blood, we have still another phase of blood poisoning. Child-bed fever and dissecting wounds are examples of this form of **septicæmia**. The symptoms usually set in within twenty-four hours and never later than the third or fourth day after the injury. There is, at first a chill or chilliness, with thirst and moderate fever, which gradually rises. Remissions and intermissions may occur. The pulse may reach 120. Stomach and bowel disturbances are common. The tongue is red around the border, but dark and dry on top. The face becomes pallid and yellowish. The mind becomes weak or delirious. Death may occur within twenty-four hours. Fatal cases usually terminate within seven or eight days.

Pyæmia is that form of blood poisoning in which the blood is contaminated by the pus producing microbes. Little particles of pus loaded with germs from a suppurating wound or ulcer enter the circulation and are carried to distant parts, where they lodge and abscesses develop. The new abscesses may form in the lungs, liver, spleen, kidneys and even in the heart and brain.

Symptoms.—The onset of this form of blood poisoning is marked by a severe chill, followed by high fever. This, in turn, is followed by profuse sweat. The chills are repeated every day or every other day. During the intervals there may be slight elevation of temperature. There is loss of appetite, nausea and vomiting. If the lungs is the seat of a new abscess there will be a cough and difficulty of breathing. If it is remembered that the first chill of pyæmia never occurs before the second week after the injury, there will be no danger of confounding it with septicæmia, which always manifests itself within the first three or four days. The irregular intermittent type of fever, with almost hourly variations, are peculiar to pyæmia, while in septicæmia there are no such fluctuations. The mind is clear and emaciation progresses rapidly. Chronic pyæmia may be prolonged for weeks and months. In acute attacks a fatal termination is usually reached within a week or ten days.

Treatment.—Blood poisoning will rarely occur if ordinary precautions are taken to use those means which are now known to prevent the infection of wounds. The antiseptic treatment of wounds has almost made blood poisoning a thing of the past in hospitals. The first step in the treatment of all forms of blood poisoning is to cleanse the wound or ulcerating surface.

The thorough evacuation of the pus from the abscesses, whenever possible, is followed with the most satisfactory results. Our old school authorities have little or nothing to offer in the way of internal medicines beyond carbonate of amonia and digitalis when the prostration is great. The same authorities recommend alcohol in large quantities. The following homeopathic remedies are often of value: **Arsenicum, Belladonna, Bryonia, China, Carbo Veg, Lachesis, Phosphorus, Rhus Tox, Veratrum Virdie.**

ANTHRAX.

This disease is also known by the names: Malignant pustule, splenic fever, charbon and wool sorters disease. It is a wide-spread disease among animals, occuring more particularly in cattle and sheep. In man it is accidental, as a result of absorption of the virus containing the germ, *bacillus anthrax*. Anthrax is the most wide-spread of all infectious diseases. While rare in America it is very prevalent in Europe and Asia. The ravages among sheep is not equalled by any other plague. Animals have been successfully protected from the disease by vaccination. The germs enter through, the skin, the intestines and the lungs. The disease is found in those whose work brings them in contact with animals or animal products.

Symptoms.—When the infection enters through the skin there is a slight itching and burning at the point of entrance. A pimple rapidly develops, on the crest of which there is a little watery blister. Under the blister there is an eroded point. The skin around this point is greatly inflamed and swollen. Other pimples and blisters form in the same vicinity. The inflammation extends to the neighboring glands and keeps on extending until the whole system is intoxicated with the poison; finally resulting in death.

in from three to five days. There is a form in which there are no pimples, but simply extensive swelling, which ends in gangrene and usually death.

The germs may enter the intestines by means of the milk and meat of animals affected with the disease. The symptoms are then those of intense poisoning. There may be a chill, vomiting or diarrhœa; also pain in back and legs, difficult breathing, livid appearance, hemorrhages and convulsions. Of twenty-five persons who ate meat infected with this disease six died within forty-eight hours.

Treatment.—The prompt cauterizing or removal of the part affected with the knife, when practical, is an approved treatment when the infection is through the skin.

Injections of ten per cent of carbolic acid about the point affected is also highly recommended. One case has been reported cured by **Lachesis.** The remedies indicated in carbuncle would likely be applicable in this disease.

HYDROPHOBIA.

This disease, belonging to animals, is frequently communicated to man by inoculation. It is more often met in the dog, wolf and cat. It may affect any of the other animals, wild or domestic. It is also known by the names of lyssa and rabies. It possesses the characteristics of other germ diseases and no doubt is caused by a bacillus.

The period between the introduction of the virus and the development of the symptoms varies according to the age, the part bitten, the extent of the wound and the animal that communicated the infection. They develop sooner in children. Wounds about the face are most serious; next those on the hands. The punctured wounds are the more dangerous. The severity depends directly upon the amount of laceration and the extent of surface afforded for absorption. The most virulent infection follows the bite of a wolf, the cat next and third, the dog. Only a small per cent. of those bitten by dogs become affected by the disease.

Symptoms.—May be divided into three stages. *Preliminary, furious* and *paralytic*. During the *first* stage there may be irritation, pain or numbness at the point bitten. The patient is depressed and gloomy. There is headache and loss of appetite. The patient is irritable, sleepless and in constant fear of something. A bright light or a loud noise is distressing. The throat is reddened and there is difficulty in swallowing. The voice becomes husky. The temperature and pulse rise but little above normal.

The *second* or *furious* stage is marked by great excitability and restlessness. The least thing will provoke a spasm of the muscles of the throat. Swallowing is so difficult that the patient dreads the sight of water. During the spasms of the throat the patient may be maniacal, but in the interval between, the mind is clear. The patient rarely attempts to injure the attendants. The second stage lasts from thirty-six to seventy-two hours, and gradually passes into the *third* or *paralytic* stage, when the patient becomes quiet, the spasms do not return, the heart's action becomes feeble, and death takes place usually on the third day and always before the seventh.

Treatment.—The best preventive is to muzzle the dogs. The wound should be cauterized with caustic potash or carbolic acid. A wash of the permanganate of potash has been recommended. We have been accustomed to use it on all wounds produced by a dog bite. Five grains put into half a glass of water will make the beautiful pink solution used so extensively as a gargle for the throat. Its disinfecting power has been proven to be very great.

Good authorities say that a genuine case of hydrophobia has never been cured. When a case becomes hopeless put the patient in a dark room with as few persons about him as possible. Chloroform and morphia are the best palliative drugs. Cocaine applied to the throat will diminish the sensibility sufficient to allow the patient to take liquid food. The Pasteur preventive treatment of rabies by inoculation has passed the crucial test and deserves to be ranked with vaccination for small-pox. Statistics show that it prevents the disease in 994 cases out of 1,000 bitten by dogs known to be mad.

There are a number of homeopathic remedies which would appear to be indicated in this disease. Chief among them is **Belladonna**, which is said to have not only curative, but preventive qualities. As soon as one is bitten, this remedy should be given in small doses every third day. **Hyoscyamus** and **Stramonium** are also indicated.

LOCK-JAW (Tetanus).

This disease is characterized by severe spasms of the muscles. It is caused by a bacillus which is found in the earth and sometimes in putrefying substances. It frequently follows a punctured wound of the hand or foot, but it may occur in persons who have received no wound. The injury is usually slight and receives but little attention at the time it occurs. The disease, as a rule, appears within two weeks after the injury. The germ that produces the disease has been identified and cultivated.

Symptoms.—The patient complains at first of a slight stiffness of the neck or difficulty in moving his jaws freely. Chilly sensations and real chills may occur. Gradually spasms of the muscles of the neck and chest produce the condition known as lock-jaw. The eyes and mouth may be much distorted. Each time the paroxysms include more muscles until all the muscles of the body are in a convulsion. Those of the back are most affected, which cause the patient to assume a hoop shape, the head and feet being drawn backward. The pain is agonizing and the patient may not be able to utter a word, the muscles of the throat being firmly set. The temperature may be elevated much or little. The mortality rate is about 80 per cent.

Treatment.—The patient should be placed in a dark and quiet place. It may be necessary to feed him by the rectum. The spasm should be controlled by chloroform. The following homeopathic remedies may be indicated: Aconite, Arnica, Arsenicum, Belladonna, Chamomilla, Ignatia, Rhus Tox, Nux Vom. and many others. Chloral has been used successfully.

SYPHILIS.

This disease, vulgarly called pox, has existed from Mosaic times and belongs exclusively to the human race. It is propagated and perpetuated by inoculation and by hereditary transmission. The point of inoculation is usually upon the privates, but may be elsewhere; lips, nipples or hands. Inoculation upon the hands is generally accidental and is a misfortune that sometimes befalls physicians in the performance of their legitimate, professional duties. Wet nurses sometimes give or receive the disease through the nipples. The most common way by which the disease is communicated is by sexual contact with one having the disease. In former times, before the day of vaccination with ivory points, the disease was sometimes communicated by means of infected humanized virus used in vaccination. Contagion from bovine virus is not possible, because animals cannot be inoculated with syphilis; even monkeys will not take the disease. The disease may be inherited from an infected father; the mother being free. It is a fact, that a woman who has borne a syphilitic child is thoroughly protected against the disease as if by vaccination. In one case, a man who has but recently had the disease may become the father of a healthy child, while in another the child may be syphilitic though the father has had no signs of the disease for years. The rule is that the longer the interval between the date of inoculation of the father and that of the birth of the child, the less likely is the child to inherit the disease. A man who has had thorough treatment and has been free from all signs of the disease for three or four years, is not likely to transmit it. A man who has symptoms of the third stage of the disease may have healthy children. A woman who has acquired the disease will likely bear unhealthy children, though the father be free. When both parents have had the disease the probability of the children inheriting it is much greater.

It should be noted that the first born are more likely to have the disease than the second or third child. We have known of an instance where the father was diseased and the mother was not. The first six children died soon after birth from hereditary syphilis, but the next six were healthy and lived. The Colles' law regarding syphilitic infection is as follows: A child born of a mother who is without obvious syphlitic symptoms, and which, without being exposed to any infection subsequent to its birth, shows this disease when a few weeks old—this child will infect the most healthy nurse whether she suckle it or merely handle or dress it; and yet this child is never known to infect its own mother, even though she suckle it while it has syphlitic ulcers on the lips and tongue.

The disease has all the characteristics of a germ disease, which it is now believed to be. There are three well defined stages of syphilis, known as the *primary*, *secondary* and *tertiary*. The first stage extends over a period varying from six to twelve weeks. With the termination of the first stage the second stage begins and continues from two to four years. The dividing line between the second and third stages is not so distinct. The duration of the tertiary stage is unlimited. It may continue twenty years.

Symptoms.—On an average, three weeks after exposure to the disease, at the point where the virus was absorbed a small red pimple forms, which gradually enlarges and breaks, leaving an ulcer consisting of a cup-shaped depression, situated upon an elevated and inflamed base. The flesh bordering the ulcer becomes hard and gristly, from whence the ulcer gets the name, hard chancre. The size of the ulcer varies and may be so small as to be overlooked; especially is this likely to be the case when it is located in the water passage.

Glands within the vicinity of the ulcer enlarge and become hard. If the chancre is upon the privates the glands in the groin will be the ones affected. If the lips be the seat of the chancre the glands beneath the jaw will be enlarged, and those under the arm; in case the ulcer is upon the nipple or hand. During this stage the general health of the patient is good and he suffers no inconvenience from the ulcer. The swollen glands are painless, a point that distinguishes the disease. The name bubo is applied to a swollen gland in the groin. The ignorant frequently pronounce the word "blue balls."

The primary stage thus being completed the **secondary** now begins, rarely earlier than six weeks or later than twelve weeks after intimate contact with one who had the disease. Unlike the primary the secondary is characterized by a number of constitutional disturbances. There may be a mild, continuous fever of a remittent type, in which the temperature reaches 101 or higher. This fever has been frequently mistaken for remittent fever. A severe headache is usually continuous with the fever. The face is either flushed or pale and jaundiced. The most pronounced symptom that marks the secondary stage is the breaking out, and which readily distinguishes the disease from all others. The eruption is variable and usually occurs on the abdomen, chest and front of the arms. The face is often free, yet we have seen it a number of times upon the forehead. The spots are reddish brown or copper colored; the color is frequently compared to that of the rind of smoked ham. The eruption may resemble measles or small-pox. Again, the rash may consist of dry scales and be mistaken for an entirely different skin disease. In the folds of the skin where there is constant moisture, there may be a thickening of the skin covered with a grayish secretion. During this stage the mouth and throat become sore. Ulcers are frequently seen on the tonsils. Sore, white patches on the border of the tongue and inside of the cheek. Warts, sometimes called fig warts, may develop at the lower orifices. There may be severe inflammation of the eyes during the secondary stage from three to six months after the appearance of the chancre. Falling out of the hair is a common symptom of secondary syphilis. As already stated the passing from the secondary to the **tertiary** stage is not sharply marked. During the latter the disease affects the deeper structures of the body. The bones and cartilages are affected. Deep ulcers occur, perforating the nasal septum, that is the cartilage between the nostrils. The roof of the mouth may be also perforated. The bones of the skull may also be partly destroyed. Running or sloughing ulcers and abscesses may develop and persist. Gummy tumors are common. Ulcers on the shin-bones, which refuse to heal, are frequently seen. Various nervous diseases may follow years afterwards. Locomotor ataxia is supposed to be a result of syphilis.

In the hereditary form of the disease may be seen all the symptoms found in the acquired except the chancre. The child may be born with well marked signs of the disease, or it may be healthy looking at birth. As a rule the latter is the case and after a month or two the disease shows itself. Hard knots in the skin about the wrists and ankles or on the feet and hands at birth indicate the disease.

In those apparently healthy at birth the disease shows itself between the fourth and eighth week by *snuffles*, causing difficulty in nursing. This may at first be mistaken for ordinary catarrh, but soon other symptoms will reveal the true character of the affection. The nasal bones may rot, causing the bridge of the nose to become depressed as if broken. The eruption occurs soon after the appearance of the snuffles and is first seen upon the buttocks. Cracks form at the corners of the mouth and ulcers in the mouth. The secretion from these sores are very poisonous. The wet nurse is very likely to take the disease from this source and other members of the family may also take it. The hair of the head or eyebrows may fall out. Children with hereditary or congenital syphilis rarely thrive and usually die early. They usually look wasted and very old. Their growth and development are slow. The disease is sometimes easily recognized by the cranial and facial appearance. A young man of twenty may not appear any more mature than a boy of ten.

The teeth have a distinctive peculiarity. The cutting edge of the tooth is narrower than the base and presents a surface like a number of pegs placed in a line. It is the upper central incisors of the permanent set which tell the story of the parentage. Inflammation and abscesses of the bones frequently occur after the sixth year. Ulceration of the shin bone is not uncommon.

Prevention.—The skillful physician can readily determine whether a case is syphilitic or not, and it is best for the patient to tell the truth, the whole truth and nothing but the truth. Barring accidental contagion it is a disease that one should be ashamed to possess. Leprosy alone is more loathsome. The disease seems to have been preordained as the penalty for promiscous sexual intercourse. It has existed from time immemorial and will probably continue to the end of time or until human nature is radically changed. The social evil and syphilis are inseparably linked together. Moral purity must ever remain the greatest preventive against both. In times of war, when morals are generally at a discount, the disease has its greatest development. A high moral and religious sentiment, along with early marriages, limits its growth in a community or nation. Young men who leave the restraints of a rural home and come to a large city have their moral stamina put to the severest test. The seclusion of a large city affords every opportunity to gratify any unhallowed desires. The person who would resist successfully all such temptations should first of all *avoid* evil associations. The easiest way to avoid these is to form good associations. The church societies afford the best and are the most accessible to a stranger in a large city. Any Christian church will welcome any young man or woman who desires the benefit of its associations.

The young man or woman who drinks stands on the brink of destruction. Drink is the gate to the social evil. Idleness affords room for lustful thoughts. Hard work, mentally and physically, is the best sedative for passion. Animal food and stimulating drinks render the passions more excitable.

The state enacts measures to protect its citizens from the ravages of small-pox and other contagious diseases, but whether it should or should not regulate the social evil so as to protect them against syphilis, is a debatable question which has strong advocates on both sides. The physician looking at the question from strictly the professional side of it would favor regulation. He knows, as no one else knows, what havoc is recklessly wrought among innocent mothers and helpless infants. In the tertiary stage the disease loses its power of being communicated to others.

Treatment.—" One night with Venus and two years with Mercury " is a significant expression when we come to consider the treatment of syphilis. Mercury in some form or other has been the favorite remedy for three hundred years for this disease, and to be effectual it must extend over a period of two years, more or less. The old school treatment is now practically limited to two drugs, mercury and iodide of potash, both of which are claimed to be specifics for it. The former is given in the secondary stage and the latter in the tertiary. The mercury is given in one grain doses from two to six times a day or a drachm of mercurial ointment is rubbed into the skin every evening for six successive days. On the seventh a hot bath is taken and on the eighth the rubbing is resumed.

A favorite prescription with the eclectics is a mixture of syrup of Stillingia one ounce to iodide of potash one drachm, taken three times a day in teaspoonful doses. Apparently good results are obtained from it when given in the secondary or tertiary stage.

On the theory that the chancre was local from the first, local means have been used, but in vain. Excision and cauterizing have proved injurious rather than beneficial. The homeopaths arrived at this conclusion in an early day. The best allopathic authorities now agree with them.

That mercury and iodide of potassium are valuable remedies in the treatment of syphilis cannot be denied, nor can it be denied that their use is frequently and shamefully abused. There are a score of homeopathic remedies that may be indicated in this disease. **Nitric Acid** is particularly useful in the so-called syphilitic sore throat which often arises from the continued abuse of mercury. This remedy is also indicated when there are gray, shallow ulcers inside of the cheeks; chancres with a tendency to bleed call for this remedy, as do also raw, moist surfaces in the folds of the skin.

In the first stage of the disease, when the chancre appears, **Mercurius Sol** is the generally indicated remedy. It ought also to be preventive. **Mercurius Iodide** is preferred by some, who claim that it will heal the chancre in six weeks and that there will be no secondary symptoms. Two grains 1x are given night and morning, first week; at night, second week; and every other day, third week. If the chancre shows a tendency to a destructive spreading **Mercurius Cor** will usually arrest its rapid progress. Hahnemann says that so long as the spot where the chancre was located has a reddish or blueish appearance the internal disease has not been cured. When the disease is completely and radically cured the location of the chancre cannot be detected. The chancre should be washed carefully with castile soap and water three times a day and lint soaked with tincture of calendula, diluted 1 to 4, should be applied after each washing. **Hepar Sulph** is another remedy that is useful after the abuse of mercury. It will hasten the suppuration of a bubo, or ripen an abscess. A flax-seed poultice will also aid and contribute to the comfort of the patient. The following remedies will at times be indicated: Phosphorus, **Ferrum**, Lycopodium, Sulphur, Silecea, **Arsenicum**, Carbo Veg, Thuya and Sepia.

The waters of various thermal springs are supposed to have a curative action upon syphilis. Prominent among these is the Hot Springs of Arkansas. Their chemical analysis would not suggest any remedial quality. But the fact remains that thousands of patients annually are cured or are benefitted at such places. The heat of the water, no doubt, has a beneficial effect in stimulating the cutaneous circulation. At all of these springs drugs are used to the best advantage. Besides, rest and change of climate always act favorably.

The treatment of syphilis and other venereal diseases affords a rich field for quacks, who flourish upon the ignorance and credulity of the thousands of poor, sinful unfortunates. It should be remembered that they have no remedies or means of treating these diseases which are not within the reach and at the command of any skillful family physician. It should not be forgotten that even in syphilis the homeopathic treatment is by far the most satisfactory in the end.

TUBERCULOSIS.

This disease may occur in several different parts of the body, but when it affects the lungs it is called consumption. Its cause was unknown until 1882, when Dr. Koch demonstrated to the world that it was due to a germ which has been named *bacillus tuberculosis*. Koch's discovery was a brilliant one and paved the way to others; in fact it solved the mystery of infectious and contagious diseases. The germs of tuberculosis are found in clusters or knobs called tubercles, hence the name tuberculosis. It is estimated that this disease is the cause of one-fifth of all deaths. It exists in all countries and in all races, and it has been known to exist from the days of the early Greek physicians. Latitude has less to do with it than altitude; it being rare on high mountains.

Indians and negroes are more susceptible to the disease than those of the white races. It prevails more in crowded cities than in rural districts. It is common among the domestic animals, especially cattle, the milk and meat of which sometimes convey the infection. The germs of the disease are everywhere. A patient in the advanced stage of consumption will expectorate in twenty-four hours from two to four billion germs. They readily attach themselves to particles of dust. The expectorations drying and rapidly becoming dust are scattered far and wide. One hundred and eighteen samples of dust were collected from hospitals, asylums and private houses where there had been consumptives. In forty of these samples the germs of tuberculosis were found, and consumption in animals produced by them. The germs grow in a number of substances, but they thrive best in the serum or watery portion of the blood, kept at the temperature of the body. They are readily taken into the lungs with the dust of the air, and if there is a disturbance of the circulation, a weakened and congestive spot from whence serum is oozing, a fertile field is ready for them. The development of tuberculosis is the natural result. Tuberculosis is not inherited as often as formerly supposed. In fact, hereditary consumption is now considered a thing of rare occurrence. The fact that it is not unusual for several members of a family to have the disease does not prove it to be inherited. It is more likely to be acquired by the intimate associations of a family. It is related that a well-to-do farmer in one of the eastern states had a large and healthy family until one of his sons married and brought home a consumptive wife. She died. Her husband was her nurse. In course of time he died also from the disease. His sister nursed him and within a year after his death she too died of the same disease. And so it went on, one member after another of the family dying until six had been buried. The night after the last funeral the father, believing that the house had something to do with so many deaths in his family, deliberately burned it, with all its contents. A new house was built, but never another death occurred in that family from consumption, though there were several members of it remaining. How and how often the disease is inherited are as yet unanswered questions. It is variously estimated to be inherited in from ten to fifty per cent. of the cases. Guinea pigs have been inoculated with tuberculosis by an apparently healthy child born of a consumptive mother. Persons who handle or experiment upon the dead bodies of those who have died of the disease, whether it be men or animals, are sometimes inoculated upon the hands. Butchers and handlers of hides are subject to local inoculation of the skin. When the disease remains local and forms reddened masses, like a cluster of inflamed warts usually seen upon the back of the fingers, hands and arms. Tuberculosis frequently occurs in the bones, joints and other parts of the body. Tuberculosis of the joints has been known in the past as white swelling, hip joint or ankle disease. All those diseased conditions known in the past as **scrofula** have been shown to be tuberculosis. Cold abscesses are usually the result of tuberculosis of the bone. Most cases of rectal fistula are tubercular. Scrofulous sores, often seen about the neck, arise from the same cause. Tuberculosis may occur in the bladder, in the testicle, or in the ovary. Potts' disease of the spine is of tubercular origin. Tuberculosis has been communicated in the following ways: Wearing the ear-rings, washing the clothes, by a bite or by a cut from the broken spit glass of a tuberculous subject.

The breath of a tuberculous patient is not infectious, though the phlegm contains millions of germs. Thousands of persons have the disease and recover. Post mortem examinations of those who have died by accident show that a large percentage of them have had tuberculosis. Statistics show that as high as 60 per cent. have had the disease. The post mortem examination of 125 infants that died at the Foundling's Home in New York found the bronchial glands tuberculous in every case.

Tuberculosis is more common in institutions where the inmates are confined and the amount of fresh air limited. In general, eighteen out of every hundred deaths are caused by tuberculosis. But statistics extending over a period of twenty-five years gathered from thirty-eight cloisters or convents, showed that 63 per cent. of all the deaths in these institutions were due to tuberculosis.

The nurses and doctors in consumptive hospitals rarely take the disease. But husbands frequently take it from wives and wives from husbands. Milk conveys the disease. The milk from tuberculous cows was fed to a number of pigs and without scarcely an exception the pigs took the disease. Intestinal tuberculosis in children no doubt often arises from infected milk. The disease is probably less frequently conveyed by infected meat, because it is generally cooked, while, as a rule, milk is taken raw. Any food supposed to be infected should be thoroughly cooked. No age is exempt from tuberculosis. During the first ten years of life the disease is more frequently found in the intestinal glands, the bones and the coverings of the brain, than it is in later years.

Catarrhal conditions are favorable for the development of tuberculosis. As already mentioned, the disturbance of the circulation affords a fertile soil for the development of the germs. And the natural resistance of the system being below par they readily develop. Pulmonary consumption often dates from a neglected cold. Tuberculosis frequently follows an injury. In such cases also the natural resistance of the body must be weakened. Inhaling impure and dusty air renders the development of the disease easier. Measles, whooping cough and exhausting fevers are often followed by tuberculosis. The weakened condition again, no doubt, facilitating its development. It is believed that the germs may be localized for years in some part and show no serious symptoms until something has depressed the nervous system, when the disease develops suddenly with great violence. It is known that the germs from a local infection may all at once be distributed throughout the entire system.

In cases of this kind, called **Acute General Miliary Tuberculosis**, the patient, after a few weeks of declining health, becomes weak and feverish. The pulse and temperature increases.

The cheeks are flushed in the afternoon, but pale in the morning. Many other symptoms, suggestive of typhoid, are present. There is but little cough. The temperature will rise to 103 in the evening and perhaps fall to nearly normal in the morning. The irregularity of the temperature distinguishes it from the steady rise of typhoid. Again, the temperature may be highest in the morning, a condition said to be more common in general tuberculosis than in any other disease. The rapid breathing and the livid skin will also distinguish it from typhoid.

In the **Pulmonary Form** of acute miliary tuberculosis there is a sudden outbreak of the symptoms pointing to marked lung trouble. The patient may have had a cough for years or have been supposed to have the disease in a chronic form. An attack of measles or whooping cough may have recently occurred. With some such antecedents as these the disease begins suddenly with the symptoms of an ordinary cold upon the lungs. The breathing is very difficult and very rapid. The cough is marked. The phlegm is mattery and sometimes rusty colored. The lividity of the skin is marked. Temperature may rise to 102 or 103. The disease proves fatal within ten or twelve days or may be prolonged for months.

The **Meningeal Form** of acute general miliary tuberculosis is known as tubercular meningitis, also known as acute hydrocephalus, or "water on the brain." In this form the tubercles filled with germs develop in the coverings of the brain, sometimes involving the spinal cord. The meningeal form is more common among children between the second and fifth year. It is usually preceded by a tuberculous condition of the lungs or of the glands surrounding the intestines.

The first symptoms of the disease are so insidious that they escape attention. It may begin with a gradual failing of health. The child gets thin, restless, peevish, irritable and loses its appetite. Its disposition is entirely changed. The disease may set in during convalescence from an attack of measles or whooping cough. Very often it follows a fall upon the head. The first striking symptoms of the disease are usually a headache, with fever and vomiting. Sometimes there will be convulsions. The pain in the head is intense. The child puts the hand to the head and sometimes gives a short, sudden cry. Again it may scream until it is exhausted. The vomiting seems to be without cause. The contents of the stomach are projected out of the mouth with such force as to carry it several feet. There is a peculiar irregularity of the breathing. In the second stage the patient becomes more quiet and all the symptoms usually subside until a stupor sets in, which usually ends in convulsions and death. This form of meningitis is considered incurable.

Scrofula is tuberculosis of the lymph glands. Material from scrofulous glands injected into Guinea pigs invariably develops tuberculosis and proves fatal within a few months.

The scrofulous form of tuberculosis runs a slower and milder course. This may be due to a feebler variety of germs. It has been said that scrofula during childhood is a sort of protection against consumption in later years; a vaccination as it were. Yet, an open scrofulous sore is very likely to develop acute general miliary tuberculosis.

A common form of scrofula called **Local Tuberculous Adenitis** is frequently met in children; especially those living in the impure atmosphere of badly ventilated lodgings. The glands under the jaw are first involved. They are frequently described as enlarged *kernels*. They may continue to enlarge and develop into an abscess, which finally breaks. The healing of the opening thus formed is usually a very slow process.

The glands about the bronchial tubes may become involved in a similar matter.

Another common form of scrofula met in children affects the mesenteric glands of the intestines, called the mesenteric form of local tuberculous adenitis. It is generally known as *Tabes mesenterica*.

The little patients are puny, wasted and bloodless. Impaired nutrition is apparent. The abdomen is large and distended. Diarrhœa, persistent. The stools are thin and offensive. There is little fever. The half starved, wasted and shriveled appearance is most striking. The disease is sometimes spoken of as consumption of the bowels, but this is not strictly correct, as it is the mesenteric glands about the intestines that are involved.

Consumption is pulmonary tuberculosis and is frequently called *Phthisis*. It is met in three forms: The acute, the chronic ulcerative and the fibriod, or hardened. The *acute* form is known as *galloping* consumption, and is met in both children and adults. It is generally precipitated by a cold or some debilitating condition. It is frequently mistaken for pneumonia, the symptoms of which it very much resembles. The fever, however, is more irregular and not so continuous as in that disease. But after the eighth or tenth day instead of a crisis occurring as in pneumonia the symptoms keep right on and even become aggravated. The sweat is profuse and the expectoration mucus and pus like. The detection of the presence of the germ, *bacillus tuberculosis*, will still perhaps be the only positive proof that the disease is consumption and not pneumonia. The case may terminate fatally within three weeks or it may be protracted three months. There is a variety of acute consumption called *acute tuberculous broncho-pneumonia*. It may attack persons apparently in good health, but over-worked or "run-down." Hemorrhage may be the first symptom. Repeated chills may occur. Temperature high, pulse rapid and breathing accelerated. The loss of flesh and strength is surprising. This form is very frequently met in children after some infectious disease as measles or whooping cough.

The Chronic Ulcerative Phthisis is the class of pulmonary tuberculosis to which the majority of the cases of consumption of the lungs belong. The germs cause tubercles to form. The tubercles decay and ulcerate. Their liquid remains are expectorated and a cavity is made. The first cavity is generally found in the right lung just below the middle of the collar bone in front. The next is located usually in a line represented by the spinal border of the shoulder blade when the right hand is placed on the opposite shoulder and the elbow elevated on a plane with the nose and opposite the fifth dorsal spine. Examination should be made, therefore, at the back as well as in front of the chest. The disease is found a third more frequently in the right than in the left lung.

The ulceration forming a cavity may destroy a blood vessel and hemorrhage, profuse hemorrhage follow. Cavities may apparently heal and remain quiet for years. Ulceration in the larynx may occur, destroying the vocal cords and causing the loss of the voice.

The Symptoms of Consumption, as commonly met, are varied and their development is gradual, even insidious at times. The dyspeptic symptoms are often prominent. The patient shows signs of dyspepsia, becomes pale and bloodless before there are any lung symptoms. Chills of a malarial type may be the first symptoms of the disease. Again it may seem to date from a neglected cold, or a hemorrhage may be the first intimation of ill health. Pleurisy may be the first suffering experienced. Of ninety cases of pleurisy with effusion thirty ended in consumption.

Huskiness or loss of voice, caused by the tubercular deposit about the cords, may be the first thing that leads the patient to consult a physician. Profuse night sweats usually occur.

The course of consumption may be divided into three periods: The first embracing the time occupied in the development of the tubercles. The second, in which they soften, and the third, in which the cavities are formed. Pleuritic pain may be an early symptom. It may be present or absent throughout the course of the disease. Cough is one of the earliest and the most constant symptom from the beginning until the end. Dry and hacking at first, but later becomes loose, when the expectoration is glaring and mattery like. There may be cases without a cough. A case may also be far advanced without any expectoration.

The first signs of consumption that can be detected in the phlegm by the naked eye are small grayish or greenish gray mattery masses. These masses should be examined microscopically. The presence of its germs is the infallible sign of the disease. It is of the *greatest importance* that a *microscopical* examination be made *early*. Hemorrhage of the lungs indicates that the disease is already well advanced rather than just beginning. The temperature is one of the most reliable indicators as to the progress of the disease. It should be taken several times a day. The temperature is usually lowest between 2 and 6 a. m., and highest between 2 and 6 p. m. During the early stage when tubercles are forming and during the period of softening there is always fever. The weighing scales is another reliable index of the progress of the disease. The weght decreases as the disease progresses.

Fibroid Phthisis is the third form of pulmonary tuberculosis. It is limited to the apex of one lung. A hardening process follows one of the other forms. The cavity becomes surrounded by dense fibrous tissue. This form is chronic, lasting from ten to twenty years, and the sufferer may enjoy fairly good health. The chest is sunken and the shoulder on the affected side is lower. In these cases the heart is often drawn out of place.

Treatment.—Any one who has read the preceding pages carefully and understands the nature of tuberculosis will at once see that it is easier to prevent the disease than to cure it. The general idea of the prevention of this disease may be summed up in a sentence: Guard against everything that is likely to weaken the natural resistance of the body. The details would require volumes. It would include protection of the feet, of the chest, of the throat, of the stomach and of every other part. Attention not to one thing alone, but to a multitude of little things which, if neglected, make inroads upon the vitality. Many cases of consumption date from a cold, or a neglected catarrh. The chief cause of catarrh is a disturbed or unequal circulation. Again we may sum up the whole matter of prevention in a single sentence: Preserve a perfect circulation, which is not only of the first importance in the prevention, but of equal value in the treatment of the disease. In many cases the disease is discovered too late to cure. But any one can soon detect any deviation from health. Treatment should begin *then*, before the disease has been determined. Change of occupation or of climate made early will do wonders. From an indoor occupation to one outside is generally highly beneficial. Bicycle riding and other out-door exercises do much to restore tone to a shattered and weakened nervous system. We know of nothing that will improve the nervous system of brain workers so much as bicycling.

Debilitate nerves are such constant and essential factors in the development of consumption that one author classes it as a nervous disease. The disease occurs less frequently in a high altitude. A large percentage of the cases of consumption are preceded by disturbances of the stomach. A good digestion is another factor of prime importance in the prevention of the disease. Many cases of catarrh cannot be cured until the stomach is put in good order. Pastry, ice cream and iced drinks are foes to a good digestion. A diet of one article of food exclusively for thirty days will almost invariably produce serious disturbances of the stomach and bowels. It is claimed that consumption of the bowels may be produced in thirty days by a diet of oat meal exclusively.

The Salisbury treatment of consumption consists f a diet of meat and hot water. A pint of hot water is drank an hour before eating the meat, which is the best lean beef prepare nic y and fairly well cooked. Absolutely no other food is allowed. Great success is claimed for his treatment.

Burt's prevention and cure of consumption by *Suralimentation of Liquid Food* consists of forcing the patient to take the greatest possible amount of liquid food. His theory is based on the fact that three-fourths, by weight, of the human body is water and that the supply of this element is insufficient in all wasting diseases.

By forcing the patient to take from one to two gallons of water by neans of palatable drinks and liquid foods he claims to be able to ncrease the weight of any patient in the first or second stage of the disease, from one-half to two pounds a week. The following are a few of the liquids he mentions as being the most common and useful in the treatment of consumption: Pure water, mineral water, Vichy water, water with tar, water with phosphoric acid, water with sugar, water with salt, carbonated water, grape juice, beer, cider, lemonade, orangeade, milk, condensed milk, skimmed milk, butter milk, pulque, wine, wine whey, scraped lean beef water, toast water, barley water, crust coffee water, clam juice, conch clam juice, fluid beef extract, extract of beef (Armour's), Valentine's meat juice. Liebig's beef tea, beet tea, egg nogg, coffee, tea, chocolate, cocoa. rice water, bread jelly, oat meal porridge, oat meal gruel, arrow root, malted milk, gum water, koumiss, lime juice, pine apple juice, strawberry juice, all fruit juices, fruit syrups, fruit jelly waters, malt extracts, and a score of other liquid preparations, consisting almost entirely of water. Our observation of this treatment has not been sufficient to enable us to say how much it will accomplish. That it will make the lean fat is quite certain. In consumption progressive emaciation is one of the positive evidences that the disease is progressing. It is also a well-known fact that abstaining from liquids diminishes the weight rapidly. Since we begun writing on this subject the champion prize fighter, Jack McAuliff, told us that when he is training for a fight he reduces his weight by abstaining, as much as possible, from all liquids of whatever kind. Many other points in matters of diet and health of equal value can be learned from the training which brutal prize fighters undergo for six weeks preparatory to a fight.

Another author, Gregg, states that the blood of a consumptive is always too watery, owing to its loss of albumen through the expectoration. He accounts for the rapid emaciation by the fact that the muscles and many other parts are developed and sustained entirely from albumen. The continual loss of albumen by the expectorations deprives them of their support and they shrink, causing the general appearance of emaciation.

Every time a mucous surface is irritated, whether by a cold, drugs or mechanical means, blood serum escapes, and it is largely composed of albumen. The germs of consumption flourish in blood serum and perhaps the reason that consumption so often dates from a cold is because the germs are first nourished and given a foothold in the escaping serum. When the mucous membrane is perfect there is nothing on its surface that will nourish the germs of consumption. But back of all, what deranges the system and causes the serum to escape so that germs can gain a foot-hold? That is the question. Deranged nerves must be the answer. Every blood vessel, every gland and every part of the body is supplied by nerves which control the action of that part. The mucous membrane is also controlled by the nerves that ramify and supply it. Then to correct any abnormal condition of the mucous membrane or any other part we must act upon the nerves. No wonder many regard consumption of nervous origin. We are, therefore, justified in the conclusion that whatever will improve the general tone of the nervous system will be of value in the treatment of consumption. Pure air, change of climate, change of occupation, change of diet, improve the condition of the nerves. The value of homeopathic remedies also becomes apparent. While, as a rule, everything will fail to cure an advanced case of consumption, we feel certain that the indicated homeopathic remedy has and will continue to arrest and prevent the disease in thousands of cases. Yes, ninety per cent. of those in the incipient stage.

It is readily seen that any remedy in the Materia Medica might be indicated, yet the following are those most commonly needed:

Arsenicum.—Wheezing respiration; cough on retiring and on rising; shortness of breath on lying down. **Baptisia,** typhoid symptoms. **Belladonna,** dry, hollow cough. **Bryonia,** cough, with stitches in the chest. Cough, with headache, as if head and chest would fly to pieces. Cough at night, compelling one to sit up at once. **Calcarea Carb,** painless hoarseness, voice hardly audible. Shortness of breath on going up the slightest ascent. Sore, pain in the chest, as if beaten. Chest painful to touch and on inspiration. Dry cough morning and night. **Carbo Veg,** painless hoarseness. Great roughness in throat. Rough voice, fails on exercising it. Desire to be fanned. **Causticum,** hoarseness with rawness. Burning and soreness in the chest. **China,** suffocative night cough, as from the vapors of sulphur. Chest sensitive to touch. **Drosera,** deep sounding, hoarse, barking cough. Must press hand on chest when sneezing or coughing. **Ferrum,** extreme paleness of the face, which becomes red and flushed upon the least pain, emotion, exertion or embarrassment; flushes easily. **Kali Bichro,** expectoration, stringy and tenacious. **Kali Carb.** cough begins at 3 a. m. Sticking pain in left chest on deep breathing. Worse, when resting. Voice, gone. Cutting pain in chest. Greenish or white masses coughed up. Weakness. **Lachesis,** hoarseness; hemorrhages; typhoid condition. Often beneficial. **Lycopodium.** See the Materia Medica, Part II. **Phosphorus,** dry, tickling cough, with tightness across chest. One of the best remedies, but must not be given too often. Some repeat the dose once in fifteen days. **Pulsatilla,** useful in lung troubles of females dating from puberty. Longing for fresh air. Down hearted.

Sulphur has perhaps cured more cases of consumption than any other remedy. For its indications see Materia Medica, Part II.

It is needless to remind the intelligent reader that all expectorations from a consumptive should be **disinfected**. Boiling water destroys the germ. So will a five per cent. solution of carbolic acid, or a one per cent. solution of bichloride of mercury. A practical way of disposing of the expectorations is to have the patient spit on a newspaper or into a Japanese paper handkerchief and then burn it. Flies may carry the infection. Spittoons are filthy and dangerous. The floors of the apartment of a consumptive should be dampened before sweeping and the sweepings should be burned.

The habit of spitting upon the floors and the sidewalk is a dangerous one, because the expectorations soon dry and become dust, to be blown and carried everywhere.

The man who marries a consumptive girl may expect to be a widower soon after the first child is born; especially is this likely to be the case if she nurses her baby, a thing that a tuberculous mother ought never to do.

DYSENTERY.

This disease, sometimes called flux, is probably an infectious disease, but the germ that causes it has not yet been fully determined. If contagious at all it is only mildly so, and in this respect it may be classed with typhoid. While it is comparatively rare in the temperate zone it is one of the four great epidemic diseases of the world, being more fatal in the tropics than cholera. It has been more destructive to armies than powder and lead. During the late civil war there were over a quarter of a million cases in the Union armies. The disease is less prevalent than formerly. Persons of all ages and of all races are subject to it. It is more prevalent during the summer and autumn. Impure water, poor food, constipation and taking cold are factors in the development of the disease. The disease consists of inflammation and ulceration of the mucous membrane of the large intestines. There are four varieties of dysentery: *Acute catarrhal, Tropical, Diphtheritic* and *Chronic.*

The **Acute** form begins with a simple, painless diarrhœa which, in the course of thirty-six hours, develops the characteristic features of the disease, namely: Colicky, griping pains in the abdomen; frequent stools, with continual straining; 'a never-get-done' sensation, called tenesmus. The constant desire to go to stool is the most distressing symptom. During the first forty-eight hours the stools are mucus, mixed with blood, but afterward they become jelly like and bloody. The movements may be very numerous, all the way from fifteen to a hundred a day. By the end of the first week the mucus becomes darker and the blood less. Grayish, thready material now passes. Mild cases run a course of eight days. Severer cases may continue four weeks. There is more or less fever at the beginning,

The **Tropical** form of dysentery is peculiar to the tropics. The onset is very much like that of the acute form. So are the stools, at first. But later, the distinguishing feature of the disease is present, namely: Liquid stools; from six to twelve yellowish gray liquid stools are passed daily for weeks. Abscess of the liver and of the lung are frequent complications of this form of the disease.

The **Diphtheritic** form of dysentery may, in the beginning, be mistaken for typhoid. The violence of the sudden onset and the bloody stools so early distinguishes it from typhoid.

The **Chronic** form of dysentery is not easily distinguished from chronic diarrhœa. There are from four to twelve movements a day. There may be constipation at times. Blood is present in the stools now and then. The ghastly appearance is striking.

Treatment.—Dysentery is another disease in which the homeopathic treatment is infinitely superior to that of the old school; especially is this true if the patient is a child. A great number of remedies may be indicated, but the following are the ones most commonly needed.

If the attack begins suddenly with a chill followed by high fever with burning hot skin and great restlessness, **Aconite** is indicated during the first stage. But as soon as the tenesmus, the never-get-done straining, with constant desire to go to stool begins, then **Mercurius Sol** is needed and will, in the great majority of cases, be sufficient to give marked relief. If the stool should now be mixed with shreds or membranes resembling the lining of the bowels, **Cantharis** is indicated. Should the disease persist after this remedy, then **Kali Bichro** is to be studied. It will be indicated by long strings of mucus. In case the discharges should become exceedingly foul and of a chocolate color, accompanied with a deathly appearance, cold skin and other signs of great prostration, **Arsenicum** is the remedy needed. But before choosing Arsenicum another remedy having many symptoms similar to it should be studied, that is **Lachesis**. Should the amount of blood be unusually great and of a dark color, then **Hamamelis** should be thought of. Pond's extract may be given in teaspoonful doses. A number of other remedies may be indicated during the course of the disease. **Belladonna, Podophyllin, Nux Vomica, Nitric Acid, Aloes** and

China are some of the more prominent ones. The last mentioned is particularly useful when the exhaustion is great, the discharges chocolate colored and the odor terribly foul. When all remedies have failed **Sulphur** should not be forgotten. Its indications are easily found in the Materia Medica, Part II.

GERMAN MEASLES.

Rubella or Rotheln is an eruptive fever which was once supposed to be a hybrid measles or a hybrid scarlet fever, but it is now believed to be a separate and distinct disease. It attacks adults as well as children. Having had measles or scarlet fever is no protection against the disease. It is contagious and spreads with great rapidity. Epidemics of it may be very extensive. The **Symptoms** develop about ten days after exposure. They are mild and there are no complications worthy of mentioning. It is a much less serious disease than either of those of which it was formerly supposed to be a species.

At the beginning there is headache, pain in head, back and legs, running at nose, chilliness and slight fever, reaching, perhaps, 100. The rash appears the first or second day, which first comes out on the face then on the chest and within forty-eight hours it covers the entire body. The other symptoms may be so mild that the rash is the first thing wrong, noticed by the mother. It usually consists of a number of round or oval slightly raised spots, pinkish in color, usually separated at first, but may run together. The color is brighter than that of measles. It remains out two or three days and leaves the skin slightly stained. There is a slight scaling off. The glands about the neck may be swollen,

The **Treatment** rarely requires more than **Aconite, Belladonna** or some other common remedy, for the catarrhal symptoms

LEPROSY.

This disease is minutely described in the XIII Chapter of Leviticus, and is supposed to be of Egyptian origin. While one of the oldest of recorded diseases, it was not until A. D. 1880, that the germ that caused it was discovered and cultivated. It was found in the tubercular like nodules on the skin. Animals will not take the disease. Baring accidental inoculation it is generally communicated through the sexual relations. It is rarely communicated otherwise. Sisters of charity have nursed them for forty years without taking the disease. In respect to its contagiousness it is very much like syphilis. It prevails extensively in hot countries. It is estimated that there are a quarter of a million of lepers in India. There are a few lepers in America, at Key West, New Orleans, New Brunswick, Nova Scotia and on the Pacific Coast, occurring not infrequently among the Chinese. There are a great many cases on the Sandwich Islands. There are 1,100 lepers in the settlement at Molokai. There are two forms of the disease, the **Tubercular** leprosy and the **Anæsthetic.**

The *first* begins with over-sensitive and sharply defined patches of reddened skin, which in time develops into nodules. The eyelashes and eyebrows fall out. The mucous membrane becomes involved. The voice fails and is lost. The throat is destroyed and death follows. The eyes may be also eaten out. Other parts may be similarly affected. The *second* form begins with pain in the limbs and spots of numbness, the opposite of the first in this respect.

Nodules soon develop in these places and break, leaving destructive ulcers. The fingers and toes may become involved and drop off. The course of this form is extremely slow. A prominent minister is said to have had the disease thirty years without impairing his usefulness.

Treatment.—No cure is known for the disease. A nourishing diet is recommended. Some one of the following homeopathic remedies would seem to be indicated: **Arsenicum, Hepar Sulph, Lycopodium, Mercurius Silicea or Sulphur.**

From time immemorial the leper has been shunned and made an outcast from society. In nearly all countries they are located in colonies or hospitals by themselves, objects of charityrity.

GLANDERS.

This is an infectious disease of the horse, which is occasionally communicated to man. It is known by the formation of nodules in the nostrils and under the skin of the horse. The germ that produces the disease resembles that of tuberculosis. It may be inoculated upon a raw surface of the skin. The symptoms develop within three or four days after the germs are deposited. It develops with fever, swelling and redness. The glands enlarge and become nodular. These may suppurate. There are pains and swelling in the joints. Abscesses may form in the muscles. The symptoms are very much like those of blood poisoning. The *acute* form runs its course in about eight days and it is generally incurable. The *chronic* form may last for months and terminate in recovery, though death by pyæmia is not uncommon. When the disease is located in the nose it is called glanders, but when in the skin it is known as farcy. The diagnosis in doubtful cases may be verified by inoculating guinea pigs. They will die within thirty hours, the testicles being found swollen and ready to suppurate. In horses a matter is discharged from one or both nostrils of a grayish or greenish color, mixed with yellow and streaks of blood and sticking like glue to the border of the nostrils. **Arsenicum, Lachesis** and **Sulphur** are the best indicated homeopathic medicines.

LUMPY JAW.

This is a chronic inflammatory affection produced in cattle and hogs by the actinomycosis or ray fungus and known by the name *actinomycosis*. It is sometimes communicated to man. The disease is usually located about the mouth and throat, hence the name, "big jaw." The disease has been classified into the *alimentary*, the *pulmonary*, the *cutaneous* and the *cerebral*, according to the part affected. The disease is often mistaken for blood poisoning. It is really a chronic pyæmia. The fever that accompanies it is like that which belongs to suppuration. Its **Treatment** is like that of pyæmia.

EPHEMERAL FEVER.

This fever, of slight duration, is sometimes called *Febricula*. Its causes are varied and its duration three to five days. The cases of ephemeral fever may be grouped according to their supposed origin. Those arising from a mild or abortive type of infectious diseases; those that are dependent upon stomach troubles as often met in indigestion of children; those caused by foul gases; those dependent upon some disturbance unrecognized. This fever begins with a slight indisposition, loss of appetite, headache, flushed cheeks and high colored urine. There may be in children a slight cough. After two or three or four days the symptoms all disappear leaving no after effects. The indicated homeopathic remedy will usually be **Nux Vomica, Aconite, Belladonna Mercurius** or **Pulsatilla.**

ACUTE FEBRILE JAUNDICE.

In 1886 Weil described an infectious disease accompanied by fever and jaundice. The disease sets in suddenly with a chill, headache, pain in the back, legs and muscles. The fever has marked remissions and lasts from ten to fourteen days. Jaundice appears early: Stools, clay colored. Liver and spleen are swollen. **Aconite, Mercurius** and **Phosphorus** are likely to be indicated remedies.

MILK SICKNESS.

This disease was quite common in the early settlement of this country west of the Alleghany mountains. It has disappeared with the clearing of the forests and is rarely found except in parts of North Carolina. It is supposed to have originated in eating the flesh and milk of diseased animals. The butter and cheese were also poisonous. The disease was severe and often fatal. The symptoms were pains in stomach, nausea, vomiting, fever and intense thirst. The tongue swollen and tremulous. Many symptoms like typhoid were present, and the odor of small-pox. The disease in cattle was known as *trembles*. The animal would stagger and all the muscles would tremble. Convulsions in animals as well as in humans frequently occurred, followed by death. While we have no record of any cases ever being treated by homeopathic remedies, the symptoms point strongly to **Gelsemium.**

MALTA FEVER.

This is a disease that prevails in Malta, Naples and other places along the Mediterranean. Its true character has not yet been determined. It has many of the symptoms peculiar to typho-malarial fever.

MOUNTAIN FEVER.

This disease is met in those residing on mountains. Whether it is typhoid or malarial is as yet an unsettled question. It not infrequently proves fatal. Study the remedies of the diseases it resembles.

SWEATING SICKNESS.

This disease is known by a fever, profuse sweat and a fine rash of blisters filled with water. From the character of the rash it is sometimes called *miliary fever.* There has been 194 epidemics in Europe during the last 160 years. Some of them were confined to a single city and continued from one to three weeks, attacking many people. The death rate was often high.

SECTION II.

Constitutional Diseases.

(*Non-Infectious.*)

RHEUMATISM.

Rheumatism is one of the most common complaints in the temperate zones, but rarely met in the tropics. Its cause has not yet been definitely determined. It has some of the characteristics of an infectious disease, but it is not at all contagious. No case of inoculation with it has ever been reported. No germ has, as yet, been positively identified with it, although an Italian physician has just claimed to have discovered one.

An over-worked or run-down condition with derangements of digestion usually precedes an attack of rheumatism. Defective nutrition and poor blood seem to be essential conditions for the disease. Lactic acid is found in excess in the blood of rheumatics. Dogs and cats injected with a solution of lactic acid die soon afterwards. Their post mortem examinations show a rheumatic inflammation of the lining of the heart. Lactic acid is a product of starchy food. In fact starchy food cannot be utilized in the body until it is converted by the process of digestion into lactic acid. A condition of the system which is unable to dispose of the excess of lactic acid thus formed is no doubt the rheumatic condition.

The chief exciting causes are dampness and suppression of perspiration due to a sudden change from a warm to a cold atmosphere. Poisonous matters that should pass off are probably retained in the system and become disturbing elements.

There are several varieties of rheumatism and different classifications by different writers. Three general forms are commonly recognized: *Acute, sub-acute* and *chronic.* Other varieties are sometimes described. The *muscular* may be classed with the sub-acute or chronic. The *gonorrhœal* is an inflammation of the membrane in one of the large joints, occurring during the course of an attack of gonorrhœa. Especially is this liable to happen if the urethral discharge has been suppressed. The *syphilitic* resembles genuine rheumatism, but is due to the poison of syphilis inflaming some of the joints. It does not, however, involve the heart and is usually limited to one or two joints, having none of the wandering character of the regular acute articular rheumatism. *Myalgia* is only the result of a strain. A group of muscles become painful to touch and on movement, the skin covering them being highly sensitive.

Acute Articular Rheumatism is popularly known as inflammatory rheumatism or rheumatic fever. Fifty per cent. of all cases of this form occur in persons between the ages of fifteen and thirty years. Persons engaged in occupations necessitating exposure to dampness and sudden changes of temperature are more liable to the disease.

Smyptoms.—Usually after exposure to cold one of the larger joints becomes painful, enlarged, hot and reddened. Soon afterwards another is affected in the same way, perhaps in a corresponding joint on the other side of the body. Other joints may become involved until nearly all the larger joints are affected. The patient cannot move without great pain. The sweat is profuse and acid The temperature may become very high, but usually ranges from 102 to 104, rising each time the disease appears in a new place. Extension of the disease to the heart is a common and serious complication. Chronic organic heart disease is often the result. The disease may affect the coverings of the heart, of the lungs, of the bowels, of the kidneys, or of the brain. Delirium in rheumatism, however, is not always a sign that the disease has located in the brain. It is more often an indication that the blood is heavily loaded with poison. If let alone an ordinary attack of acute rheumatism would continue about six weeks. Relapses are not uncommon. One attack renders the person more susceptible to another.

Sub-acute Rheumatism is also called *muscular* rheumatism. The coverings of the muscles are involved. Any movement of the affected part is, therefore, painful. The disease may be confined to a group of muscles. For instance, the muscles of the neck, when it is known as *wry-neck*, or those of the back, when it is called *lumbago*. The suffering from this form of rheumatism often varies with the weather, being worse a few hours before a storm. No elevation of temperature accompanies it. It is most commonly met in those who have had their feet or hands in cold water for a long time. For instance, scrub women, window and carriage washers.

Chronic Rheumatism usually results from repeated attacks of acute rheumatism. Several of the joints remain enlarged, stiff and painful. Sometimes the disease comes on steadily without any really acute attack. The pain is more severe at times, varying according to the weather. The muscles, as well as the joints, are usually involved. The muscles about the affected joints become wasted. The disease may affect the coverings of the nerves as well as those of the muscles, in which case the disease is known as *rheumatic neuralgia.* There is usually tenderness in some particular spot and pain on motion. The use of the various joints affected are always impaired. Certain spinal affections may be accompanied with enlarged and displaced joints but not so many joints are involved as in chronic rheumatism.

Treatment.—In no other disease is the poverty of old school treatment so apparent. Salicylate of sodium has not proved the specific that they thought it would a few years ago. However, we must confess that we have seen great temporary relief follow the giving of half a dozen five grain powders of this drug four hours apart. Cod liver oil has been used for a century as a remedy for chronic rheumatism in old persons. Hot salt baths are beneficial in all forms of rheumatism. We have just read of cases of acute rheumatism speedily cured by ice cold applications to the hot and inflamed joints. Liniments and various applications, as a rule, do but little good and often no doubt drive the disease to the heart.

The homeopathic treatment is usually more satisfactory in the end. Relapses sometimes occur which are very stubborn. We recall distinctly a case of relapse where a celebrated homeopathic professor had treated the case with brilliant success until the relapse. But afterwards he could make no impression upon the disease. He was discharged from the case and his successor cured it with a single prescription of salicylate of sodium.

A disturbed digestion is a factor in the production of rheumatism and its correction is an important measure in its cure. The diet should be changed completely. Many so called rheumatic pains can be cured by drinking, before each meal for a month, a pint of hot water with a little salt in it.

Several homeopathic remedies may be indicated in rheumatism. In the muscular variety, caused by getting wet, **Rhus Tox** stands at the head of the list. It is particularly indicated when there is great restlessness at night. Better by motion and worse before a storm. **Bryonia** is indicated in acute rheumatism when the joints are swollen, red and hot. The patient is worse from motion. Just the opposite of the indications for Rhus tox. The thirst is great and the sour sweat profuse. **Aconite** may be very useful in the beginning, when the fever is high and the pain is severe. **Arsenicum** is strongly indicated when the patient is pale, pinched, thirsty and relieved by hot applications. **Belladonna** may be useful if there are sharp, tearing pains, coming and going suddenly. The tincture or the twelfth dilution of **Chamomilla** often gives great relief from the intense pains. It also soothes the great irritability of temper. One cheek red and the other pale is another good indication for its use. **Lycopodium** may be needed when there are present its characteristic symptoms as found in the Materia Medica, Part II. **Mercurius, Nux Vomica** and **Pulsatilla** are sometimes indicated. **Sulp'ur** is one of the most commonly needed remedies in chronic rheumatism, or when there are repeated relapses of the acute form. **Phytolacca**, the polk root, is also a valuable remedy in chronic rheumatism, as well as an effectual agent in reducing superfluous fat.

ACUTE GOUT.

This affection characterized by paroxysms of pain is thought to be due to an excess of uric acid in the blood. It occurs chiefly in those of sedentary habits who indulge to an excess in the luxuries of the table; especially of meats, sweets, sweet wine and malt liquors. Those who have ceased an active, out-door life for a sedentary one without any change from their former heavy diet, are liable to the disease. The tendency to gout is hereditary and the disease may affect one strictly temperate in all things. An attack may be brought on by any unusual excess, by a fit of anger, by worry or by exhaustion. It may come on without any warning, again it may be preceded by indigestion, irritability and despondency. An attack usually sets in at night. The patient, who is always over thirty years of age, is awakened by severe pain, which is located in the joint which unites the big toe with the foot. There is fever. The pain moderates toward morning and the patient falls asleep, again to be disturbed in a similar way the succeeding night. The joint becomes tender, red, swollen and puffy. The skin finally peels off. Other smaller joints may become involved. The attack gradually subsides, leaving the affected joints somewhat stiffened and swollen. At the height of the attack the amount of uric acid in the blood is increased, while that of the urine is diminished. But as soon as the attack is over the normal amount is again passed off with the urine. The disease may leave the joints suddenly and affections of the stomach, heart or brain follow.

Chronic Gout usually results from repeated attacks of the acute form of the disease. Chalk like deposits, consisting of urates, take place about the affected joints. These deposits may be formed in the lobe of the ear, in the kidneys, in the spleen, and also in the walls of the smaller blood vessels.

Treatment.—First of all, the lazy, gluttonous habits must be abandoned. A light vegetable diet and abundant regular exercise in the open air must be taken. In the acute form the following homeopathic remedies may be indicated: **Aconite, Arnica, Arsenicum** and **Bryonia.** In the chronic form the main remedies are **Sulphur, Calcarea Carb, Lycopodium** and **Silicea.** The remedies indicated in rheumatism may be studied to an advantage.

LITHÆMIA.

This affection is a modified form of gout. The urine contains an excess of uric acid and urates, also phosphates and calcium oxalate in superabundance. The urine is scanty and passed frequently with a burning sensation. Cramps in the legs, eruptions on the skin, noises in the ears, disturbances of vision, palpitation of the heart, cough, headache, dizziness, drowsiness and despondency, are some of the many symptoms that occur in this disease. There is also a sallowness or an unnatural redness of the complexion. The appetite is poor, the taste metallic, the digestion deranged and the bowels constipated. This disease is frequently mistaken for other troubles. It usually terminates in an incurable disease of the kidneys and heart.

Treatment.—A careful attention to diet and a study of the Materia Medica in Part II will do much to arrest the progress of this disease, if not indefinitely postpone its worst features. A meat diet should be avoided.

ARTHRITIS DEFORMANS.

This affection, properly called rheumatoid arthritis, and improperly called rheumatic gout, is a destructive disease, involving both large and small joints. It is accompanied with deformity, impaired mobility and pain. The cartilages uniting the bones become absorbed. The ends of the bones become enlarged and hardened. They elicit a grating sound on being rubbed together. When it affects the fingers they are usually drawn away from the thumb. The disease usually comes on slowly. Only occasionally attended with acute febrile symptoms. It occurs in the exhausted, the poorly fed, the debilitated and those whose surroundings are unhealthy. The very opposite conditions of those affected with gout. It differs from rheumatism in that it affects the smaller joints as well as the larger. In fact it may affect any and all the joints of the body.

Treatment.—Improvement of the surroundings and a better diet are the first essentials. A cure can hardly be expected. But relief may be obtained from **Calcarea Phos.** or some of the remedies usually indicated in rheumatism.

DIABETES MELLITUS.

The first sign of this disease that usually attracts attention is the increase in the amount of urine passed. A chemical examination of which, reveals the presence of sugar. Through some derangement of nutrition the sugar accumulates in the blood and is excreted in the urine. A tendency to the disease may be inherited. It is more often met in men than in women, and in those over thirty years of age. It seldom occurs in young persons. The disease is chiefly confined to the intellectual and the highly nervous. Just previous to the beginning of diabetes the patient is often very fleshy. Gout, syphilis and malaria are supposed to be some of the exciting causes of the disease. Mental shocks and worry often precede it. Injuries of the brain and spine have been followed by diabetes.

Symptoms.—The onset of the disease is gradual. The frequent passing of water, the great thirst, the voracious appetite and the immense quantity of urine, varying from six to forty pints a day, are the prominent symptoms. The specific gravity of the urine is always greater than the normal, ranging from 1025 to 1045. The color is pale and looks very much like pure water. Analysis shows from one to ten per cent. sugar. In spite of the enormous amount of food eaten the patient, as a rule, becomes rapidly emaciated. The skin is dry and harsh, rarely perspiring. Boils and carbuncles are common complications. The patient is often annoyed by eruptions and intolerable itching. Gangrene is not an uncommon complication, while lung troubles are frequent. Various nervous disorders are found complicating the disease.

Treatment.—The diet is an important part of the treatment. If carefully followed out according to the rules below, all cases will be benefitted if not cured. The patient may take the following liquids: Oxtail, turtle, bouillon and other clear soups, coffee, tea, chocolate, cocoa and lemonade. No sugar must be used in any of them. Saccharin may be used instead. Soda, potash, apollinaris vichy water and milk may be taken.

Of animal foods the following are allowed: Fish of all sorts, salt and fresh, poultry and game, eggs, butter, buttermilk, curds, cream cheese and all fresh meats except liver. The only bread allowed is gluten and bran bread, also almond and cocoanut biscuits. The starchy foods must be avoided. White bread being perhaps the best example of that class. The vegetables allowed are lettuce, tomatoes, spinach, chiccory, sorrel, radishes, water-cress, mustard, celery and pickles of various sorts. Lemons, oranges and currants are allowed, also nuts.

The following must be avoided: Thick soups, liver, crabs, lobsters and oysters; ordinary bread, including rye, wheaten, brown, white and all such articles, as rice, tapioca, sago, arrow root and vermicella. The following vegetables are prohibited: Potatoes, turnips, parsnips, squashes, beets, corn and asparagus, also beer, sweet wines and sweetened drinks. The main point to keep in mind is that all sugar producing foods must be avoided. Perhaps fifty homeopathic remedies may be indicated in as many diabetic cases. To mention any one or two remedies would be misleading. One must study the Materia Medica, Part II.

DIABETES INSIPIDUS.

Diabetes Insipidus is an entirely different disease from *diabetes mellitus*. About the only resemblance between the two is that in both an immense quantity of urine is passed. In the former the specific gravity of the urine is too low, ranging from 1001 to 1009, while in the latter it is too high, ranging from 1025 to 1045, or even higher. The urine in the former contains no sugar nor, as a rule, any other abnormal element, while that of the latter is loaded with sugar, the characteristic feature by which we recognize the disease. The former is more frequently met in young persons, while the latter is rarely met in persons under thirty years of age. The former is a much less serious disease than the latter. Diabetes insipidus is supposed to originate in some derangement of the nervous system.

It often follows a fright or an injury. There are other diseases in which a large amount of urine is passed of low specific gravity. But in each case it will contain some abnormal element that will distinguish it from the urine of diabetes insipidus.

Treatment.—The cause must be removed if possible. Cold drinks should not be taken in large quantities. There are no routine remedies. **Apis, Belladonna** and **Phosphoric Acid** are sometimes indicated. Each case must be given remedies according to the symptons.

RICKETS.

This is a disease belonging to infants. It is known by the impaired nutrition and by the alterations in the bones. It is found in all parts of the world, but chiefly among the children of the poor, who have been deprived of sun light and of pure air. Too much starchy food, too much cow's milk and poor feeding generally are important factors in the development of the disease. The bones of richitic children contain only about one-third as much lime salts as they should.

Symptoms.—The disease comes on slowly, rarely before the sixth month or after the second year. Digestive disturbances, fever, restlessness, irritability and sleeplessness, are usually present. The child is so sensitive all over that it cries whenever it is moved. There is such profuse sweating during sleep that the pillow is wet for some distance about its head. The bones are soft and yielding. The sides of the chest yield so that the "pigeon breast" is formed. Nodules form where the ribs join the breast bone. The ends of the long bones become enlarged, while their shaft bends, as in case of the "bow legged." The head appears large and the open spaces in the skull, natural at birth, are tardy in closing. Teeth decay early and fall out. The abdomen is often enlarged, giving rise to the so-called "pot bellied." The spine may be curved. The disease is never in itself fatal, but such children do not resist well other diseases.

Treatment.—The child should have the best food and the purest air. If it is still nursing the health of the mother or nurse should receive the most careful attention. The child should be given other food besides that which it nurses. Cow's milk properly diluted along with strained oat meal gruel is a good addition to its diet. Bovinine, a beef preparation that may be procured at any drug store, is of great value in such cases. The child should be rubbed night and morning with olive oil or cod liver oil. The chief homeopathic remedies are **Calcarea Carb** and **Calcarea Phos.** Other remedies may be needed, such as **Belladonna, Sulphur, Lycopodium, Sepia** or **Silicia.**

SCURVY.

This affection, sometimes called scorbutus, is known by the great debility, the anæmia, the spongy gums and the tendency to hemorrhages that attend it. The disease has been known from the earliest times. It was formerly common among soldiers in the field and among sailors on a long voyage. But since its cause was discovered, during the early part of the present century, it has become a rare disease. The disease develops in those who have been for a long time deprived of fresh vegetables or their substitutes. All agree that the disease is caused by an absence in the diet of the salts which vegetables possess. The disease is now occasionally met only in poor houses, lumber camps, mining regions and other places where vegetables are not obtainable. Depressing influences and unhygienic surroundings are believed to favor the development of the disease. The most recent striking instance of the occurrence of scurvy was among the prisoners at Andersonville during the civil war.

Symptoms.—The disease comes on slowly. The patient loses in weight and steadily grows weaker, also paler. The gums become swollen, spongy and bleed easily. The teeth loosen and may fall out. The breath is foul and the tongue swollen. The skin becomes dry and rough. Very small black and blue spots appear first on the legs and then on the arms and trunk. The slightest bruise or injury causes hemorrhage into the part injured. Nose bleed, hemorrhage from lungs, stomach, bowels and kidneys are not uncommon. The heart palpitates. The soreness of the gums prevents the patient from eating much. Constipation is more often present than diarrhœa. The urine often contains albumen. Its specific gravity is high and the color deep.

Treatment.—A correction of the diet will speedily cure the majority of the cases of scurvy if not too far advanced. The juice of two or three oranges daily, with plenty of fresh vegetables, will usually be all the treatment necessary. Some cases will require one or more of the following homeopathic remedies: **Arsenicum, Carbo Veg, China, Mercurius, Natrum Mur, Nitric Acid, Nux Vom., Phosphorus** or **Sulphur.**

PURPURA.

This term indicates a condition where there are black and blue spots in the skin produced by hemorrhages in the skin. The spots may vary in size from a pin head to the size of a silver dollar. The small ones are called petechial and the larger ecchymoses. At first they are bright in color, but become darker and finally fade, leaving a brownish stain. This condition occurs with a number of diseases. As septicæmia, pyæmia, malignant endocarditis, typhus fever, measles, small-pox. It also occurs after snake bite, poisoning by certain drugs, as belladonna, mercury, quinine, ergot, iodides and copaiba. It is seen in Bright's disease, scurvy, Hodgkin's disease and in the aged, especially about the ankles and wrists. It may be seen in cases of locomotor ataxia, where there are lightning pains, and in other neuralgiac troubles.

Purpura hemorrhagica is a severe form of the disease in which hemorrhages take place from the mucous membrane. When the disease is associated with rheumatic symptoms it is called *Purpura rheumatica*. Simple cases recover in a week or two, but those in which there is considerable hemorrhage may be variously complicated and protracted.

Treatment.—Improve the diet and surrounding conditions. The following homeopathic remedies should be studied: **Phosphorus, Arsenicum, Arnica, Bryonia, Lachesis** and **Hamamelis.**

HÆMOPHILIA.

This is a hereditary tendency to uncontrollable hemorrhages. The slightest wounds bleed profusely. Their tendency to bleed has been traced in some families through several generations. In the majority of instances the hemorrhage occurs from the nose. It may continue for hours and even for days. The younger the person is when the disease manifests itself the less the chances of outgrowing the tendency. Of 152 boys with this weakness 81 died before the end of the seventh year of age.

Treatment.—Phosphorus is the best indicated homeopathic remedy for this trouble. **China, Ferrum, Arsenicum** and **Hamamelis** may be of service.

SECTION III.

Diseases of the Digestive System.

STOMATITIS.

This is an affection of the mouth and manifests itself in six forms, *Acute, Aphthous, Ulcerative, Parasitic, Gangrenous* and *Mercurial.*

Acute stomatitis is sometimes called catarrhal, from the fact that it is a catarrh of the mucous membrane of the mouth, resulting from irritation by something taken into the mouth or by a decayed tooth. It is known by the increased secretions, the unnatural redness and heat. Taking food into the mouth causes discomfort. The appetite is poor and the breath foul. The tongue may be swollen, furred and indented.

Aphthous stomatitis manifests itself at first by little blisters on the inside of the cheek, the border of the tongue and on the inner surface of the lips. These break and leave small, grayish ulcers with bright red borders. It is more frequently seen in children under three years of age. It develops rapidly and may disappear almost as quickly. It must not be confused with *thrush*, which is the **Parasitic** stomatitis and is produced by a fungus parasite, belonging to the yeast family. Poor food, uncleanliness of the mouth, acid fermentations arising from remnants of food lodged in the mouth favor the development of parasitic stomatitis. It is not infrequently communicated by unclean spoons and nursing bottles. We meet this form not only in children suffering from stomach and bowel troubles, but in adults in the last stage of consumption or diabetes. It first appears on the tongue in the shape of raised pearly white patches, which run together and spread to other parts of the mouth. These patches can easily be scraped off and leave no ulcer beneath, as is the case in aphthous stomatitis. The mouth is dry, the opposite of the condition met in the acute form of stomatitis.

Ulcerative stomatitis is also known by the name, *putrid sore mouth*. It prevails in jails, camps and institutions with unhealthy surroundings. Poor food, lack of cleanliness of the mouth, decayed teeth, collection of tartar on the teeth favor the development of the disease. It spreads like an infectious disease. Some maintain that this disease and the foot-and-mouth disease of cattle are one and the same. It begins at the margin of the gums, which become red and swollen, bleeding easily. Ulcers form along the gum lines of the upper and lower jaw, covered with a grayish white membrane. There is a profuse discharge of saliva, the breath is foul and chewing is difficult. The glands beneath the jaw enlarge. A wash of chlorate of potash is said to be almost a specific for this trouble.

Gangrenous stomatitis, also called *cancrum oris* or *noma*, is a gangrenous process which starts on the gums or cheek and rapidly destroys the surrounding tissues, burrowing a hole perhaps into the jaw or perforating the cheek entirely. This rare but terrible disease is only met in children with unsanitary surroundings or in those convalescing from some acute fever, especially measles. The sufferers are usually between the ages of two and five years.

Mercurial stomatitis is the result of poisoning by mercury. It is sometimes called *Ptyalism*, on account of the profuse flow of saliva from the mouth. It was formerly very common in the days of heroic doses of mercury, but this cruel treatment, along with bleeding and many other barbarous methods, has been banished since the advent of homeopathy. The unfortunate victim of salivation by calomel first complains of a metallic taste in his mouth, the gums swell and become red and sore. The tongue is also swollen, the breath foul and the teeth loosen, sometimes falling out.

Treatment.—Each one of the six forms of stomatitis just described requires different treatment. Perfect cleanliness of the mouth is the first essential. Careful attention to the diet and the surroundings are the next. Washing out the mouth with borax and honey is an old domestic remedy not without merit. A modern preparation, Listerine, diluted to one-fourth or more, is an excellent mouth wash. It renders the mouth clean and sweet. Soap suds, made of the purest soap, is an effectual wash. The following homeopathic remedies are frequently indicated: **Nux Vom., Sulphur, Mercurius, Nitric Acid, Hepar Sulp. and Baptisia.**

PTYALISM.

This affection is an excessive secretion from the salivary glands. It is met in a number of diseases; certain mental and nervous troubles, hydrophobia, small-pox and in some other acute diseases. It is very common during the earlier months of pregnancy. It is readily produced by a number of drugs, chief among these are mercury, gold, copper, iodine, jaborandi, muscarin and tobacco. Unless produced by them the following remedies are useful: **Mercurius, Nitric Acid, Ipecac, Arsenicum, Belladonna.** When there is an insufficient secretion of saliva the condition is called **Xerostimia**, and has been cured by electricity; galvanic current. The parotid glands, located on both sides between the ears and the angle of the jaws, sometime inflame as in mumps. The condition is called *Parotitis*. It is often produced by mumps, but sometimes by other diseases, as typhoid, pneumonia, pyæmia. In which case, if an abcess forms, it is regarded as an unfavorable symptom.

DISEASES OF THE THROAT.

The following are the chief affections of the throat: (1). Those arising from *circulatory disturbances* including *hyperæmia, hemorrhage* and *oedema*. The hyperæmia, indicated by simple redness, may be due to the irritation of tobacco smoke or a result of organic heart disease, which causes the blood to engorge the blood vessels, giving them a bluish shade. The hemorrhage is usually due to some local cause in the throat. The oedema is generally associated with a debilitated condition of the system as found in Bright's disease. The palate and other parts of the throat have a puffy appearance. (2). *Acute pharyngitis* is *sore throat* proper. It is also called *angina simplex*. It involves the tonsils and the entire throat; usually results from cold, but may arise from various constitutional or digestive troubles. The patient complains of dryness, tickling and soreness on swallowing. If it extends down to the vocal cords hoarseness results. This form usually disappears within a short time. (3). *Chronic* pharyngitis is usually the result of repeated attacks of the acute form. It is very common in those who drink and smoke and in those who use their voice much, as clergymen. It often results from chronic catarrh. (4). *Ulceration* of the *pharynx* may be divided into six classes: (*a*) Follicular, such as come from chronic catarrh. (*b*) Syphilitic. (*c*) Tuberculous. (*d*) Pseudo membraneous, as, for example, the diphtheritic. (*e*) Fever ulcers, such as occur in typhoid. (5). *Acute infectious phlegmon* of the *pharynx* is a throat trouble in which there is much swelling, fever and a rapidly forming abscess. (6). *Retro-pharyngeal abscess* sometimes follows one of the fevers and is often the result of decay of a spinal vertebra just back of the throat, in which locality it is usually found. (7). *Angina Ludovici* is a cellulitis or inflammation of the neck that is sometimes seen in diphtheria and scarlet fever.

TONSILLITIS.

This is an inflammation of the tonsil. There is an *acute* and a *chronic* form. There are two varieties of the acute, namely, the *follicular* or *lacunar* and the *suppurative*. The first variety is more frequent between the ages of ten and thirty years. Exposure and unhygenic surroundings favor its development. Defective drainage and sewer gas are supposed to be exciting causes. It begins with a chill or chilly sensations, and aching in the back and limbs. The fever rises rapidly and may reach 105 in the evening of the first day. There is soreness of the throat and difficulty in swallowing. The tonsils are red and creamy mucus is seen in their crevices. One tonsil alone may be affected or one after the other. If both tonsils are attacked at the same time the disease will be found to arise from some poisoning. The tonsils may be so swollen as to touch each other. The fever usually subsides within a week. Tonsillitis often precedes rheumatism.

Tonsillitis and diphtheria are often mistaken for each other. To determine one from the other is often a matter of great importance. In tonsillitis the tongue is coated and furred, while in diphtheria it is, as a rule, clean. The patches in the former are cream colored, while those of the latter are a dirty gray. In the latter case it tends to spread, while in the former it does not. The fever does not, as a rule, rise so rapidly in diphtheria. When the membrane of diphtheria is scraped off it leaves a raw or bleeding surface. Such is not the case in tonsillitis. In diphtheria there is usually a swelling of the glands of the neck seen and felt externally.

The **Suppurative Tonsillitis** is commonly called *quinsy*. The cause and symptoms are very much like those of the acute form. The suffering is more intense, the saliva is more profuse and the tonsils more swollen. Within two to four days they become filled with pus and will "break" if not anticipated with the knife. Early lancing of the abscess will save the patient much suffering.

Treatment.—The indicated homeopathic remedy given early will do much toward relieving or cutting short an attack of tonsillitis. No doubt but that abscesses may be and are frequently prevented by homeopathic treatment. Salicylate of sodium is said to relieve the pain. The chief homeopathic remedies are **Aconite, Apis, Belladonna, Mercurius, Hepar Sulph., Lachesis** and **Kali Bichromicum.** The last mentioned remedy will be of great service in cases where there is much tenacious saliva stretching out into long strings. **Belladonna** is perhaps more frequently indicated. **Sulphur** may be of great service when convalescence is slow.

Chronic Tonsillitis is associated with a chronic enlargement or hypertrophy of the tonsils. This condition in children may affect greatly their mental and physical development, by establishing in them the evil habit of *mouth breathing*. The form of the chest and the expression of the face are changed by this habit, which is more noticeable at night when the child is asleep than during the day. If the mouth breathing continues for a long time the child develops a dull, stupid expression. Even the mind and disposition may become unnatural from this cause. The mental faculties and the power of attention are actually weakened. The breath of mouth-breathers is always foul. Little cheesy masses are frequently pressed from the tonsil. If they be crushed between the fingers a very foul odor is emitted. The tonsils, when perfectly normal, are scarcely visible. Enlarged tonsils are easily seen. A nasal voice is usually associated with them.

Treatment.—There are cases where amputation of the tonsil is justifiable. It is not usually a painful or serious operation. But careful and prolonged homeopathic treatment will generally render such radical measures unnecessary. One of the most effectual remedies in reducing enlarged tonsils is **Baryta Carb.** Some, however, claim that **Baryta Mur.** is even better. A dose twice a week should be given for several months. **Calcarea Phos.** is another remedy frequently indicated. So is **Mercurius Iodide.** Patients with enlarged tonsils will often exhibit symptoms calling for **Calcarea Carb** or **Iodide.** When all other remedies have failed **Sulphur** will often produce good results. **Phosphorus. Phytolacca** and **Lycopodium** should also be studied in the

Materia Medica in Part II. If the stomach is kept in a good condition by proper diet and by drinking before each meal a cup of hot water in which there is a little salt, and if the skin is kept in a good condition by a cold sponge bath every morning before breakfast, throat troubles will be of rare occurrence.

DISEASES OF THE ŒSOPHAGUS.

The esophagus or gullet may be affected as follows: (1). *Inflammation* resulting from catarrah, chemical poisoning, hot liquids, diphtheria and other irritations or diseases. There may be a great deal of inflammation in the gullet without any symptoms. In severe inflammation there is usually pain on swallowing and a constant dull pain beneath the breast bone. (2). *Spasms* of the gullet occur in hysteria, hypochrondria, chorea, epilepsy and especially hydrophobia. The patient complains of inability to swallow food and even liquids. But a bougie may be readily passed without meeting any obstructions. (3). *Stricture* of the esophagus may follow the swallowing of corrosive sublimate, the healing of an ulcer or from some mechanical pressure, as a tumor. (4). *Cancer* of the esophagus is not an uncommon disease. It is usually located in the upper third of the tube. The earliest symptom of this affection is difficulty in swallowing, which increases along with rapid emaciation. A person over fifty years of age with these symptoms, along with enlargement of the glands of the neck, has cancer of the gullet. (5). *Rupture* of the gullet may occur from severe or prolonged vomiting. (6). *Dilatations* and *Diverticula* may develop in the esophagus. They may follow a narrowing of the tube. The food lodges and the walls bulge until a sac or diverticulum is formed.

DISEASES OF THE STOMACH.

Affections of the stomach are classified as follows: *Acute gastritis, Chronic gastritis, Neuroses, Dilatation, Peptic ulcer, Cancer* and *Hæmatemesis.*

Acute Gastritis, also called simple gastritis, acute gastric catarrh and acute dyspepsia, is a common complaint and is usually caused by errors of diet. The fault of the diet may be that the food is unsuitable or too great in quantity, or it may be partly decomposed when eaten, or it may arise from drinking alcoholic liquors. Acute gastritis occurs at the beginning of many of the infectious diseases. The most common symptoms of this form of gastritis are headache, depression, nausea, belching, vomiting and an uncomfortable feeling in the abdomen. In severer forms there may be a chill and slight fever; tongue coated, breath foul and frequent vomiting. The duration of an attack is but a day or two. There are the following varieties of acute gastritis: (1). *Phlegmonous* gastritis or acute *suppurative* gastritis, a rare disease in which there is suppuration in the sub-mucous layer of the stomach. (2). *Toxic* gastritis, the most severe form of inflammation of the stomach, is caused by swallowing some concentrated acid or a strong alkali or some other poisonous substance, as arsenic, phosphorus or corrosive sublimate. The symptoms are pain in the mouth, throat and stomach, along with vomiting, in the matter of which there is blood. An examination of the inside of the mouth will usually reveal effects of the poisoning. In case of poisoning by acid, magnesia should be given in milk or white of egg. In case the poisoning is produced by an alkali then a dilute acid is the remedy.

(3). Diphtheritic or membraneous gastritis occurs in diphtheria and a number of other diseases. (4). *Mycotic* or *parasitic* gastritis is due to a fungus.

Chronic Gastritis, also called *chronic dyspepsia* or *chronic catarrh of the stomach*, is that condition of the stomach in which there is an increase in the mucus, a change in the gastric juice and an impairment of the muscular coats of the stomach so that food lies in the stomach longer than it should. The following are some of the causes of chronic gastritis or dyspepsia: Unsuitable or poorly prepared food; the continued use of certain articles of diet, as too much fat, coffee, tea and alcohol; eating at irregular hours; eating too rapidly; insufficient mastication; drinking ice water during meals; also the use of tobacco. The disease may develop as a result of the debilitating effects of other diseases.

There are two forms of chronic dyspepsia, *simple chronic* gastritis and *sclerotic* gastritis. The symptoms of chronic gastritis vary much, but the following are those usually met: Appetite, variable; feeling of distress or oppression after eating; painful feeling when the stomach is empty; heart burn; pain on pressure over the stomach; tongue, coated; bad breath; tip and border of tongue very red; saliva, profuse; morning nausea; much belching of gas; bitter fluids come up with the belching; vomiting of food immediately or an hour or two after eating, the matter vomited containing abnormal acids, such as butyric, acetic or lactic, while hydrochloric acid is entirely absent or present in a quantity much less than normal. The bowels are constipated, the head aches and the patient is depressed and constantly out of sorts. Dizziness and melancholia may occur in severe cases. The heart palpitates and there may be a cough, but no fever. Chronic gastritis is now worse and now better and may continue indefinitely unless cured. It is the unsuspected cause of many other troubles.

Treatment.—The first step in the successful treatment of chronic dyspepsia is to ascertain, if possible, the cause and remove it. In many cases the cause will be found to be over-eating or rapid eating. Another very common cause is bad cooking. On no other subject of equal importance is there so much ignorance. To be a good cook should be regarded as one of the finest accomplishments that a woman can acquire. Bad cooks cause more suffering than all the saloon-keepers in the world. For the further consideration of the subject of cooking the reader is referred to the Chapter on Dietetics. Some severe cases of dyspepsia will do well upon an exclusive milk diet. The milk being diluted one-half by soda water, vichy water or plain water, to a cupful of which has been added five grains of carbonate of soda or a pinch of salt. Skimmed milk or buttermilk will agree with many cases for awhile. Patients may even gain weight on an exclusive milk diet. Six to eight ounces should be taken every three hours, making three to five pints within twenty-four hours. In many cases it will not be necessary to limit the patient so strictly. It may be necessary only to cut off hot bread, fried articles of food, pies, cakes and other pastry. Ice cream, sweets and fats should be avoided. Toasted bread, not scorched, but toasted to a golden yellow, and brown bread are easily digested. Fruit should be eaten only in the morning before eating anything else. Again, dyspeptics must not get the idea that everything they eat will hurt them. Moderate exercise, a visit to the country or mountains, or a long sea voyage will work wonders for dyspeptics. Over-work, mentally and physically, are important factors in the production of dyspepsia. Food will not digest readily when the body is tired out or the mind worried. Proper rest of body and freedom from worry must be obtained in all cases before a cure can be expected.

Many cases will be benefitted by a cold sponge bath before breakfast, especially flatulent dyspepsia. Injections of one to three quarts of warm water, slightly soapy, every other night will relieve the coated tongue and foul breath in many cases. Peroxide of hydrogen diluted to one-fourth and taken into the stomach will destroy the fermentation and improve the condition greatly.

A cup of hot water, to which has been added a teaspoonful of bi-carbonate of soda, will chemically sweeten the stomach. Bad cases of chronic catarrh of the stomach have been promptly cured by repeatedly washing out the stomach. Teaspoonful doses of glycerine have also cured cases of this kind.

As already mentioned, hydrochloric acid is usually absent or deficient in all cases of chronic dyspepsia. One hundred drops of the dilute hydrochloric acid taken a quarter of an hour after meals is said to act well. Salt is an essential factor in the development of hydrochloric acid. The use of salt in dyspepsia has, therefore, a scientific basis.

The writer has found, by personal experience, the observance of the following two rules an excellent way of not only curing, but of preventing chronic gastritis: (1). Before each meal drink a cup or two of hot water, to which has been added a little milk, sufficient to color it well, and a pinch of salt. (2). During meals and for three hours afterwards drink absolutely nothing. If, after observing these rules, you should suffer from thirst, it is evidence that you have eaten too much or of improper food.

During the last few years it has been discovered that many dyspeptics have some abnormal condition of the rectum, especially the last inch of the bowel, consisting either of piles, or ulcers, or fissures, or stricture. The correction of such troubles is usually followed by the happiest results. A large number of homeopathic remedies may be useful in dyspepaia. The most important ones are the following: **Arsenicum, Nux Vomica, Pulsatilla, Lycopodium, Carbo Veg, Podophyllum, Sepia, Bryonia, Hydrastis, China** and **Ipecac.**

Neuroses of the stomach are included in three classes: *Gastralgia* or *gastrodynia, Nervous dyspepsia* and *Nervous vomiting.* In case of simple gastralgia not associated with any organic disease the patient is suddenly seized with severe pain at the pit of the stomach, which passes backwards and around the lower ribs. Attacks come on regularly without any reference to food. Pressure upon the stomach usually gives relief while it is continued. Eating often relieves the pain. This affection generally occurs in nervous women who are worried and constipated. More often met in those passing the "change of life."

Nervous dyspepsia has oppression and distress after eating, as in cases of chronic gastritis, but the food digests in the proper time. If the stomach is found empty seven hours after eating an ordinary meal of soup, bread and meat, the case is one of nervous dyspepsia. There are three types of nervous dyspepsia. (1). The secretions are normal. (2). They are not sufficiently acid. (3). They contain an excess of acid.

Nervous vomiting is due, not to any derangement of the stomach itself, but to nervous influences. The patients are, as a rule, female brunettes of a hysterical nature. A peculiarity of the vomiting in such cases is the absence of straining. Without effort or gagging the mouth is filled with the contents of the stomach. *Peristaltic unrest* is common in neurasthenia. Shortly after eating an annoying gurgling sound occurs which may be heard at a distance. *Rumination* is a rare affection in which the food is regurgitated and chewed, as seen in cattle. This is only met in nervous, hysterical persons, epileptics and idiots. A careful study of the homeopathic Materia Medica will detect the indicated remedies for all these. Orificial surgery, massage, electricity, bicycling and the rest cure may all be utilized to advantage in this class of stomach troubles.

Dilatation of the stomach may be either an *acute* or a *chronic* condition. The acute is rarely seen, yet it occurs whenever a large quantity of food and drink has been quickly taken into the stomach. Chronic dilatation may be due to a stricture at the pyloric outlet of the stomach, or it may be caused by simple weakness of the muscles produced by repeatedly over-filling the stomach. In chronic dilatation the vomiting of enormous quantities is the most pronounced symptom. The quantity may amount to three quarts, consisting of food and liquid. There are also many dyspeptic symptoms.

Peptic Ulcer may be present for months in the stomach without any other symptoms than those common to dyspepsia. The first positive symptom may be a perforation or a sudden hemorrhage from the stomach. In case of peptic ulcer vomiting does not occur for two hours after eating. The gastric juice is excessively acid. In one-half of the cases there is hemorrhage. The vomiting of bright red blood strongly suggests ulcer. Pain is the most constant symptom of ulcer. It may be a burning, gnawing pain, or it may come on as intense paroxysms of gastralgia. Attacks generally come on about fifteen minutes after taking food. A circumscribed tenderness is another common symptom. **Kali Bichrom.**, **Lycopodium** and **Arsenicum** are the most frequently indicated homeopathic remedies in case of ulcer of the stomach.

Of all cases of cancer one-fifth are found in the stomach. Three-fourths of the patients with cancer of the stomach are over forty years of age, while the majority of those with ulcer of the stomach are under forty. **Cancer of the stomach** may exist and even cause death without exhibiting any positive symptoms by which it could be detected. However, the following general symptoms when combined in one case strongly suggest the disease: Aggravation of previous dyspeptic symptoms; a steady, progressive emaciation; a loss of strength from month to month; a sallow, bloodless complexion; a tumor in the stomach; continued and diffused pain in the stomach, accompanied by vomiting and slight hemorrhages; the coffee-ground vomit; the continued absence of hydrochloric acid from the secretions of the stomach. The invariable presence of hydrochloric acid in the secretions of the stomach is positive evidence of the absence of cancer.

Treatment.—Cancer of the stomach is incurable. Such patients do best on a milk diet. Washing out the stomach regularly gives relief. Life may be prolonged by a surgical operation, making a new channel between the stomach and the bowels.

Hemorrhage of the stomach, also called *Hæmatemesis* and *Gastrorrhagia*, may arise from different causes. Hemorrhage of the stomach and hemorrhage of the lungs are distinguished as follows: In the former there will be found previous stomach trouble; in the latter previous lung trouble. In the former the blood is vomited; in the latter coughed up. In the former it is acid, dark colored and mixed with food, while in the latter the blood is alkaline, frothy and bright red.

Treatment.—Hemorrhage from the stomach as well as hemorrhage from other parts may be controlled by tying a cord tightly about a leg or arm or both.

DISEASES OF THE BOWELS.

The following diseases of the intestines are associated with diarrhœa: *Catarrhal Enteritis, Enteritis in children, Diphtheritic* or *Croupous Enteritis, Phlegmonous Enteritis, Mucous Colitis* and *Ulcerative Enteritis.*

Among the *primary* causes of enteritis or diarrhœa may be mentioned: Improper food; poisons; change of weather; changes in the secretions; nervous or mental influences. Among the *secondary* causes are found: Infectious diseases; neighboring inflammations; disturbances of circulation; conditions accompanying some of the incurable diseases. It should be remembered that diarrhœa is not always produced by catarrh of the bowels; mental disturbances may cause it. On the other hand catarrh of the bowels may sometimes exist without diarrhœa.

If the catarrh is in the small intestine the diarrhœa will be less profuse, the pains, colicky, and the stools, yellowish, green or grayish yellow, with particles of food and but little mucus. If the catarrh is confined to the large intestine, the pain is either absent or very intense, the stools are of a uniform consistency like soup and have a grayish granular appearance, often containing much mucus. Tenesmus, that is straining at stool, indicates that the rectum is involved. Catarrh of the bowels may be acute or chronic. An attack of the former may last from two to ten days, during which time there may be four to twenty stools within twenty-four hours. If a very great quantity is evacuated within a short time fainting or collapse may occur. The chronic form may follow the acute or may develop independently.

Enteritis in Children embraces three forms: (1). The acute dyspeptic diarrhœa. (2). Cholera infantum; and (3). Acute entero-colitis. Diarrhœas of children can almost invariably be traced to improper feeding. Hot weather and unhealthy surroundings aggravate them. In a case of the first form the child, apparently well, has an increased number of natural stools for a day or two, after which they are more frequent, offensive and contain curds and undigested food. This form may set in abruptly and violently with high fever, vomiting and griping pains. Convulsions may occur. The stools are grayish or greenish yellow. They are never watery, as in cholera infantum. The attack is generally brought on by eating unripe fruit or by drinking tainted milk. Recovery, as a rule, soon takes place, but relapses may occur and the third form develop. In case of *cholera infantum* the vomiting is incessant and is excited with every attempt to take food or drink. The diarrhœa is uncontrollable. The stools, frequent and profuse; very thin and watery. At first very offensive, but later odorless and alkaline. The eyes are sunken, the features pinched, and the complexion ashy. The tongue is dry and red, while the thirst is insatiable. Death may occur within twenty-four hours from the beginning of the attack. The child may linger in a stupor. Convulsions may occur. The head may be drawn back and the respirations may be irregular, as in brain trouble. The symptoms of a child with cholera infantum and those of an adult with cholera asiatica are almost identical.

Acute Entero-colitis is the form of diarrhœa that occurs in children after an attack of an infectious disease. It may follow the first form, or it may develop in artificially fed children any time of the year, but especially during hot weather. The stools usually contain mucus streaked with blood and are passed without pain. An attack lasts from two to six weeks. Cases of this kind may be more severe and are sometimes called acute dysentery.

In case of *Diphtheritic Enteritis* patches or a membrane resembling that seen in the throat during an attack of diphtheria form on the lining of the bowel. This condition usually follows some infectious disease, or incurable disease, as pneumonia, typhoid, pyæmia, cancer or Bright's disease.

Phlegmonous Enteritis is the name given to the condition when pus forms beneath the lining of the bowel. It is most frequently seen when the bowels are telescoped or in cases of obstruction or strangulated hernia. The symptoms are much like those of peritonitis.

Mucous colitis is a remarkable affection of the large intestines, in which long strings of tenacious mucus are passed. It may form a cast of the bowel. Attacks are commonly brought on by worry and may continue from one to ten days, attended by severe pain. On account of the severe pain the disease has been called *mucous colic*. It has also been called *membraneous* enteritis and *tubular* diarrhœa.

Ulcerative enteritis includes not only the ulcers of tuberculosis, syphilis and typhoid, but the following forms of ulceration: *Follicular ulceration, stercoral ulcers, simple ulcerative colitis, ulceration from external perforation, cancerous ulcer and solitary ulcer.* Considerable ulceration may take place in the small intestine without diarrhœa, while a small spot of ulceration in the large intestine may be accompanied by frequent stools. As a rule, however, diarrhœa is present in all cases of ulceration of the bowels. Small quantities of pus, shreds and blood are the most positive symptoms of ulceration. Large quantities of pus passed at a time would indicate that it was formed in some other organ and not in the bowel. Profuse hemorrhage also indicates ulceration of the bowel.

Treatment of Bowel Troubles.—In the successful treatment of all intestinal complaints attended by diarrhœa, two rules must be religiously observed. (1). The patient must be put to bed and kept mentally and physically quiet. (2). The patient must abstain from all food, taking absolutely nothing but water until the diarrhœa ceases. This last rule applies more particularly to acute cases, including typhoid. Patients can easily go a week without taking food. In the cure as well as in the production of bowel troubles the diet plays a most important part. Certain foods tend to constipate, while others have an opposite effect. Boiled milk, as a rule belongs to the first class, while meat and fruits usually loosen the bowels. In many, some one article of food is the sole cause of the diarrhœa.

In chronic diarrhœa with mucous stools injections of large quantities of warm water are often beneficial. In case of infantile diarrhœa during hot weather a warm bath and a carriage or boat ride into fresh, cool air will accomplish wonders. A trip to Lincoln Park or a ride on Lake Michigan has saved thousand of Chicago children during hot seasons. During the memorable heated spell in July, 1887, a three days' sail on Lake Michigan, we are positive, was the only thing that saved the eldest son of the authors. Children with acute diarrhœa should be given plenty of water, but little or no food; certainly no food as long as there is vomiting. Splendid results are often obtained by washing out the child's stomach, also from washing out the bowel. The following rule may be observed to advantage in some cases: If the stool is alkaline and has a very foul, decayed odor, give no albuminous food, of which the white of the egg and lean meat are the best examples. Give, instead, milk, sugar, crackers, oatmeal gruel, barley water and other cereal preparations. But if the stool is acid, simply sour and not particularly offensive albuminous food may be given; bovinine, meat broths and egg preparations will prove beneficial. Beef juice may be obtained by pressing fresh steak, rare and chopped, in a lemon squeezer. Beef juice thus obtained and the white of eggs are two very nourishing articles of food that are more readily assimilated than any other.

The homeopathic materia medica is particularly rich in its resources for the successful treatment of bowel troubles. The results that have attended the homeopathic treatment of bowel troubles of children are strikingly brilliant. We could readily mention fifty useful remedies for these troubles, but the following are most commonly needed: Aconite, **Arsenicum**, Belladonna, Chamomilla, Calcarea Carb, **China**, Gelsemium, Ipecac, **Mercurius**, Podophyllum, **Pulsatilla**, Rhus Tox, Sulphur and **Veratrum Alb**. The particular indications for each may readily be found in the Materia Medica, Part II.

Dilatation of the colon or large intestine may occur and no evacuation take place for two or three weeks.

Infarction of the bowel is caused by blocking of some of the terminal blood vessels of the mesentery. Severe pain, nausea and vomiting of contents of bowel accompany it. It is the usual cause of colic in horses. Fatal results may follow this as well as dilatation.

APPENDICITIS.

Where the small and large intestines unite there is a fish-worm like appendage from three to six inches long and of the size of a goose quill, which is called the Appendix Vermiformis. It is hollow, being closed at one end, while the other empties into the large intestine. It sometimes becomes the receptacle of apple seeds, shot and similar bodies, composed of dried intestinal matter. These develop inflammation, abscess, ulceration and perforation, in this part, upon slight provocation, as getting feet wet and cold. Especially is it likely to occur in persons under twenty years of age. Sixty per cent. of all cases occur in persons under thirty years of age and eighty per cent. in males. General peritonitis, resulting in death, is a common sequel of appendicitis or inflammation of the appendix. The disease is indicated by sudden pain and circumscribed tenderness in the region just above the right groin. The center of the area of tenderness will be found at the middle point of a line drawn from the naval to the point of the hip. All the region just above the right groin will have a hard, rigid feel. The disease was formerly called typhilitis and perityphilitis, but these terms are going out of use. About ten per cent. of all cases prove fatal. Many cases are saved by promptly opening the abdomen and letting out the pus. This new operation is universally approved by the best surgeons. Many cases, however, get well of their own account. An ice bag laid over the tender spot is highly recommended. In one case we are satisfied that a mustard plaster was beneficial. In another case, treated successfully, we applied a towel wrung out of cold water and had it reapplied as often as it became dry. **Aconite, Bella-**

donna and Bryonia were the indicated remedies in these cases. The great danger in these cases arise from the breaking of the abscess into the peritoneal cavity, so that the pus comes in contact with the outside covering of the gut which is peritoneum and causes peritonitis. The importance of prompt surgical interference is plain.

Intestinal obstruction may be caused by strangulation, telescoping, knots, twists, strictures, tumors and foreign substances. *Strangulation* is the most frequent cause of acute obstruction. *Intussusception* or telescoping is that condition where one part of the bowel slips into another, as the parts of a spy-glass slide into each other. *Twists* and *knots*, called *volvulus*, are the results of a loop of the bowel turned upon its axis.

Strictures and *tumors* may arise from various causes. *Abnormal contents* may consist of the following foreign bodies: Fruit stones, coins, needles, pins or false teeth. A mass of worms or a gall stone may cause an obstruction. Articles swallowed by children rarely cause any trouble. The three principle symptoms of acute obstruction are constipation, pain and vomiting. The pain comes early; at first colicky, but it becomes continuous and very intense. Severe and incessant vomiting soon follows. The contents of the stomach are first vomited, then greenish matter and soon afterwards a brownish black liquid, having a fecal odor. In case of *chronic* obstruction the symptoms are similar, but slower in developing and less violent, but may terminate fatally. Purgatives should never be given in a case of suspected obstruction of the bowel. Washing out the stomach is highly beneficial. **Belladonna** and Lycopodium may be indicated in some cases. Injection of a large quantity of water is recommended, also inflation by forcing air into the bowel by a bellows or a valve syringe. If these measures fail to give relief by the third day a surgical operation is the next and last resort.

Constipation may be constitutional or it may be produced by sedentery habits, certain kinds of food, or other diseased conditions. Inattention to the desire to go to stool is also a cause. An effort to move the bowels should be made every day at the same hour. This habit should be inculcated into children at an early age. A large percentage of cases of constipation are caused by an improper diet and may be corrected by eating laxative food. A cup of hot water with salt in it before breakfast tends to relax the bowels. Ripe, juicy fruit, eaten before breakfast, has the same tendency. Hot water salted and a juicy apple before breakfast have cured scores of cases of obstinate constipation. Dilatation of the rectum, the removal of papillæ and ulcers that are often present in the rectum, generally cures constipation. Massage of the abdomen is also effective. A cold sponge bath over the abdomen stimulates sluggish bowels. A metal ball, weighing from four to six pounds, rolled over the abdomen for five or ten minutes every morning, is beneficial. Injections of warm water are less harmful than purgative medicine. The **Constipation** of children is generally due to some fault of the diet. Often the child does not receive sufficient water. Every child, no matter how young, should be given plenty of cool water several times a day. Constipation in an infant often indicates that its food is insufficient. A teaspoonful of glycerine injected into the bowel, whether adult or infant, will usuallly cause an evacuation within three minutes, especially if the lower part of the bowel is constipated.

A large number of homeopathic remedies may be beneficial in

constipation. Remedies prescribed for other conditions often correct the constipation. The following may be studied: **Belladonna, Bryonia, Nux Vomica, Pulsatilla, Lycopodium, Opium, Sepia** and **Sulphur.**

DISEASES OF THE LIVER.

The liver may be deranged as follows: A condition often occurs producing jaundice or icterus; derangement of its blood vessels are met, also affections of the bile passage, including catarrhal jaundice and gall stone; cirrhosis or hardening of the liver may take place; abscess may form; new growths or tumors may develop; the liver may become fatty, hence the term fatty liver; or it may become waxy or lardaceous when it is called amyloid liver. Our limited space will not permit us to give a technical description of each one of these affections.

Catarrhal Jaundice is indicated by the white of the eyes and the skin turning to a lemon yellow. In case of permanent obstruction of the bile duct of the liver these become olive-green or a bronze color. The urine, sweat and saliva are also sometimes colored. A terrible itching may accompany jaundice. The stools are pale in color on account of the absence of bile in them. Pulse, often very slow. *Icterus neatorum* is a jaundice of new born infants. The mild form is natural while the severe form may prove fatal before the second week. **China, Belladonna, Mercurius, Podophyllum** and **Phosphorus** will usually cover the symptoms of simple catarrhal jaundice.

Gall Stones are calculi formed in the gall bladder. They may attain an enormous size. Three-fourths of the cases of gall stones occur in women. They are present in one-fourth of all women over sixty years of age. Tight lacing is supposed to obstruct the free flow of bile. **Biliary** or gall stone colic is due to the passing of a gall stone from the gall bladder. The most intense pain is felt in the right side at the lower border of the chest. The pain also extends to the shoulder and to the pit of the stomach. There is a chill and fever. The patient rolls in agony. There is vomiting, profuse sweat and great prostration. Attacks vary greatly in duration. As soon as the stone escapes from the narrow channel the severity of the attack suddenly ceases. Relief is obtained sometimes by having the patient drink a pint of olive oil. **China** and **Belladonna** are the most serviceable homeopathic remedies during an attack of gall stone colic. Recently many cases of gall stone have been successfully treated by removing them by a surgical operation.

Cirrhosis or hardening of the liver may be caused by alcoholic liquors, malaria, syphilis, tuberculosis, scarlet fever, rickets, heart disease, anthracosis or from coal dust. The most striking symptom of cirrhosis of the liver is the ascites or dropsy of the abdomen, which occurs rather late in the disease. The earlier stages may show no positive symptoms of any kind. The disease is incurable.

Abscess of the liver is more common in the tropics and warmer climates. It may occur in any climate as the result of an injury or of pyæmia.

New Growths in the liver may be cancer, sarcoma or angioma. Of internal cancers that of the liver is third in order of frequency, the womb, first; the stomach, second, and the liver, third. Cancer of the liver is often preceded by cancer in some other part.

When the liver is enlarged and nodular and there is jaundice, along with a pale, sallow complexion and rapid emaciation, it is probably cancerous. Although cancer of the liver may exist without any of these symptoms.

DISEASES OF THE PANCREAS.

The following abnormal conditions may occur in the pancreas: Hæmorrhage, acute hæmorrhagic pancreatitis, chronic pancreatitis, pancreatic cysts and cancer. The diagnosis of these various obscure conditions requires rare skill.

DISEASES OF THE PERITONEUM.

The peritoneum is a shut sac composed of serous membrane which lies over, around and between the intestines and other abdominal organs. It is very similar to the pleura, which is also a shut sac of serous membrane lying between the lungs and the walls of the chest. Of itself the peritoneum rarely, if ever, develops disease, but it is a fertile soil for diseased germs. They grow in it more rapidly and more luxuriantly than in any other part of the body. Pus germs frequently escape into it from neighboring abscesses; as from abscesses in the ovary, in the appendix or in other neighboring organs. Diseased germs may also be conveyed into the peritoneum through a wound, as in case of gun shot, or in case of a surgical operation in which the abdomen is opened. Within six hours after pus germs have entered the peritoneum the most violent inflammation may take place, called **Acute General**

Peritonitis. Its beginning is generally signalled by a violent chill and severe pain in the abdomen. The pain is general and is aggravated by motion or pressure. The patient lies with thighs drawn up and shoulders elevated. As a rule, the greatest pain is below the naval, but it may be above in case the pus came from an organ above the naval. Coughing and talking, even breathing, aggravates the pain. The abdomen becomes enormously distended. The pulse ranges from 110 to 150 and the temperature from 104 to 105. In no other disease, except cholera, are the features so pinched and deathly. Death may occur within thirty-six hours from the beginning of the attack, but it more commonly takes place the fourth or fifth day. There is a **Localized Peritonitis** and also a **Chronic Peritonitis.** Their names are sufficiently descriptive for the purpose of this volume. **Belladonna** and **Arsenicum** are the most serviceable remedies in acute general peritonitis. These remedies may be given in a low potency and frequently; 3x and half hourly. **Aconite** and **Bryonia** may be indicated. We have seen great benefit from applying and re-applying to the abdomen a heavy towel wrung out of ice water. It lowers the temperature, soothes the patient and seems to check the rapid, destructive progress of the disease. Clothes wrung out of hot water and upon which a few drops of turpentine have been placed, are frequently used with benefit. Turpentine is a powerful disinfectant.

Tuberculosis and **Cancer** may occur in the peritoneum and develop peritonitis.

Ascites or dropsy is the accumulation of fluid in the peritoneal cavity. It may arise from local troubles or it may be due to disease of the heart, of the lungs, of the liver, or of the kidneys. The treatment of ascites depends somewhat upon its cause. Infusion of **Apocynum**, also infusion of **Digitalis,** taken in teaspoonful doses every six hours, give temporary relief from the dropsy. Cathartics also give relief.

Diuretin is a new drug that extracts the water from the system very rapidly. It requires seventy-five grains a day to be effective. The strictly homeopathic remedies usually indicated are **Arsenicum, Apis, Bryonia, Kali Carb** and **Sulphur.** All remedies frequently fail and tapping, a simple, comparatively painless operation, is the only source of relief. Patients with ascites may live for months and years and be tapped a hundred times, relieving them of barrels of water.

SECTION IV.

Diseases of the Respiratory System.

DISEASES OF THE NOSE.

The nose may be subjected to the following affections: *Acute Coryza*, commonly called "catarrh" or "cold;" *Chronic Nasal Catarrh*, including the three forms of rhinitis; simplex, hypertrophica and atrophica; *autumnal catarrh* or hay fever, and *epistaxis* or nose bleed. The word catarrh is derived from two Greek words and literally means "flowing down." Any mucous membrane in any part of the body is in a catarrhal state when its excretions are excessive. Catarrh cannot exist without a derangement of the circulation and the rational method of treating catarrh must always include all means tending to improve the circulation. The circulation is controlled by the nervous system. Whatever impairs or improves the nervous system affects, likewise, the circulation. Direct irritation of the mucous surface is a common cause of catarrh. The irritation may be either from dust or from germs. If the skin and bowels are kept in a good condition catarrhal troubles are less likely to occur. A cold sponge bath before breakfast does much to prevent catarrh. If salt be added to the water the bath will be still more beneficial; it will decrease the chances of taking cold. Many cases of catarrh are due to stomach trouble and cannot be cured until the stomach is put in a normal condition. Acute coryza or catarrh is usually of only a few days duration, while the chronic may continue indefinitely unless cured. In the chronic form the nostrils feel obstructed and the individual must breath through the mouth. After sleep the mouth and throat are extremely dry. Chronic catarrh of the nose may affect seriously the hearing. In the treatment of catarrh homeopathy is particularly rich in remedial resources. A long list of useful remedies occurs to us. The most common ones are **Aconite, Belladonna, Arsenicum, China, Nux Vomica, Sanguinaria, Kali Bichrom, Pulsatilla, Mercurius** and **Sulphur.**

Autumnal Catarrh or hay fever comes on late in the summer with symptoms of a cold. There is also bronchitis, cough and asthma. It is not unusual for attacks to recur every year on the same day of the month. The presence in the atmosphere of the pollen of flowers or of hay is supposed to be an exciting cause. The disease has sometimes been called rose fever because the odor of roses often brings on an attack. It is related that a lady was seized with an attack by being offered an artificial rose. It is more frequently met in those highly educated than among the illiterate. It is believed to have a nervous origin.

Epistaxis or nose bleed may arise from local or constitutional causes. A blow, or picking the nose, may cause it. It frequently occurs during typhoid, diphtheria, pneumonia and other severe diseases, also when the menses are suppressed. In the majority of cases the bleeding ceases of its own accord. Yet cases of persistent bleeding may occur and demand treatment. It may be necessary to plug the nose from behind. This is accomplished by first passing a catheter, with its eye threaded, through the nostril from the front to the back. One end of the thread is caught and brought through the mouth while the other is withdrawn with the catheter. To the end of the thread protruding from the mouth a cotton plug is tied and then drawn into the mouth and up into the nostril from the back part of the throat.

If the indicated homeopethic remedy be given it will rarely be necessary to resort to plugging. The following may be studied in the Materia Medica, Part II: **Ipecac, Belladonna, China, Aconite, Nitric Acid, Carbo Veg, Phosphorus** and **Hamamelis.** Pond's extract is a reliable preparation of hamamelis and should always be thought of in case of a hemorrhage from any part. The simplest method of arresting nose bleed is to hold the arms above the head, or tie a cord about the arm, or apply ice to the nose or back of the neck. A door key hung down back of the neck is another domestic remedy.

DISEASES OF THE LARYNX.

The following affections may be found in the throat: *Acute catarrhal laryngitis, chronic laryngitis, œdematous laryngitis, membranous laryngitis,* or croup, *spasmodic laryngitis, tubercu- lous laryngitis* and *syphilitic laryngitis.*

Acute Catarrhal Laryngitis is to the throat what acute coryza is to the nose; while chronic laryngitis corresponds to chronic nasal catarrh. Acute laryngitis may arise from cold, irritating gases, over-use of voice, injury, hot liquids or poisons. It is indicated by a tickling in the throat, irritated by cold air and by breathing. There is a dry cough with change of the voice; at first husky, but later it may be lost. **Chronic Laryngitis** usually follows the acute. Over-use of the voice is a common cause. It may also result from the inhalation of irritating gases or tobacco smoke. The voice is hoarse or lost and there is a frequent desire to clear the throat. **Œdematous Laryngitis** is a puffy or dropsical like condition of the throat, due often to some other disease. It may develop rapidly and within an hour or two result fatally. The breathing is difficult and has a sawing sound. Two eminent men in their prime have died of this disease within a few months. Both suffocated. If tracheotomy had been performed no doubt both would have been saved. Better still, if both had been given **Apis** the result, we feel sure, would have been quite different. **Membranous Laryngitis** is now generally conceded to be true diphtheritic croup. A strong membrane forms in the throat filling up the upper part of the windpipe, which often produces death by suffocation or blood poisoning. The affection begins insidiously and is often mistaken for an attack of acute laryngitis; there is hoarseness and a rough cough, known as "croupy cough." After two or three days these symptoms become sudden worse, usually at night. Paroxysms of difficult breathing occur, but later the difficulty in breathing is constant. The voice is husky at first, but later it is only a whisper. As the air passage of the throat becomes narrower the color of the lips, face and finger nail become bluish, as in suffocation. The child tosses in vain for air. The upper part of the membrane can usually be seen by looking into the throat. It has a dirty gray appearance, as the ordinary diphtheritic patch. The disease usually attacks children between two and five years of age. The treatment of membraneous croup by tracheotomy and intubation is discussed under the heading, Diphtheria. **Apis, Kali Bichromicum** and **Spongia** should be carefully studied when treating cases of true croup.

Spasmodic Laryngitis, also called laryngismus stridulus, is the condition where the child seems to hold its breath until the face is congested and then there is a relaxation; the air entering the lungs with a high pitched, crowing sound. There is no cough. **Spasmodic Croup** is very similar to the affection just described. It is the false croup while membraneous laryngitis is the true croup. The child goes to bed apparently well, but awakens about midnight or a little later with oppressed breathing and a harsh, croupy cough. The symptoms of suffocation may be alarming, but the attack soon passes off and the child rises in the morning as if nothing had happened. **Aconite, Spongia** and **Hepar Sulph.** are the only remedies needed. A hot bath or an emetic is beneficial in some cases.

Tuberculous Laryngitis is due to tuberculosis of the throat and its first indication is a slight huskiness of the voice, followed by hoarseness and entire loss of voice.

Syphilitic Laryngitis may be inherited or acquired. The history of the case and the accompanying symptoms make the detection of this trouble comparatively easy for the skilled physician.

DISEASES OF THE BRONCHI.

The following affections belong to the bronchial tubes: *Acute bronchitis, Chronic bronchitis, Bronchiectasis, Bronchial asthma* and *Fibrinous bronchitis*. Like that of the nose and throat the mucous membrane of the bronchial tubes are subject to an acute and a chronic catarrhal condition. The former is called **Acute bronchitis** and the latter chronic bronchitis. The former is a common result of a cold and often is no more than the extension downward of an acute nasal catarrh or coryza. It is often called "cold on the chest." It may occur with measles, whooping cough, typhoid, malaria and some other diseases. It is accompanied with a sense of oppression of the chest and tightness or rawness under the breast bone. The cough is rough and rasping. The chest is sore and the paroxysms of coughing cause great distress. The cough is dry at first, but later loose. There may be slight fever, the first week. The natural course of the disease covers a period of two or three weeks. In children and in cases of measles or whooping cough, there is danger of broncho-pneumonia developing and terminating the case fatally. The broncho-pneumonia is indicated by very difficult breathing and by a livid color.

The habit of taking quinine to "break up a cold" cannot be recommended. Turkish baths, while beneficial, are attended with a risk of taking more cold. The homeopathic remedies, **Aconite, Arsenicum, Belladonna, Bryonia** and **Phosphorus**, secure the best results. It is our personal experience that **Ferrum Phos., Kali Mur.** and **Kali Carb**, given in the order named, invariably cut short attacks of acute bronchitis. **Aconite** and **Ferrum Phos** are particularly beneficial in the bronchitis of children.

Chronic Bronchitis may follow repeated attacks of the acute, but is more commonly a complication of other diseases, especially of the heart, lungs and kidneys. The general health may be good and there may be no distress, except occasionally. The cough is variable, changing with the weather. It may entirely disappear during the summer season and return with its usual severity as soon as cold weather sets in. A warm climate the year round is especially suited for such cases. In some cases there is no expectoration, but usually it is abundant. Homeopathic remedies given according to the general indications can and do accomplish much toward curing such cases. Those mentioned for acute bronchitis should be studied.

Bronchiectasis is a dilated condition of the bronchial tubes, due to a weakening of their walls. This condition may occur independently or in connection with other diseases. A symptom peculiar to this condition is that the patient may pass a whole day without coughing and then a sudden paroxysm come on, during which an immense quantity of phlegm is coughed up. The term, **Bronchial Asthma,** has been applied to difficult breathing, accompanying a number of diseases not connected with the lungs. The term, cardiac asthma and renal asthma, are sometimes used. The former expressing the difficult breathing occurring in heart disease and the latter that in diseases of the kidney. The term, bronchial asthma, should be limited to difficult breathing arising from an affection of the bronchi alone. Asthma and hay fever resemble each other in many points. And it is maintained that the only real difference is in their location. Asthma is sometimes hereditary It is more common in men than in women. A great many things may bring on asthma; anger, dust, strong odors, over-eating or a change of weather. A person may be free from it in one part of the country and suffer greatly in another. A change of residence is generally beneficial. There is no doubt but that it is of a nervous origin. Many cases have been cured by orificial surgery; correcting the diseased condition of the lower orifices of the body.

Asthmatic attacks usually occur during the night. The patient finds himself unable to breath, with great oppression of the chest. The face is pale, even livid, and the expression is anxious. In very severe attacks there may be cold sweat upon the forehead, a rapid pulse and cold extremities. Attacks may last from a few minutes to several hours. **Arsenicum** often gives prompt relief. **Fibrinous Bronchitis** is a rare affection, in which a tough membrane forms a cast of the bronchi and is coughed up during a paroxysm of difficult breathing.

DISEASES OF THE LUNGS.

The following derangements or affections of the lungs may occur: *Disturbances of the circulation*, embracing active and passive congestion, also œdema and hemorrhage. *Pneumonia, Chronic Interstitial Pneumonia, Broncho-pneumonia, Emphysema* including the three forms: Compensatory, hypertrophic and atrophic, *Gangrene, Abscess, Pneumonokoniosis* and *New growths* or tumors.

Congestion of the lungs may be active or passive and arise from a number of causes. The chief symptoms of active congestion are chill, fever, cough, pain in the side and difficulty of breathing. These symptoms are identical with those of the first stage of pneumonia. We have no doubt but that a prompt relief of congestion of the lungs often prevents pneumonia. **Aconite, Belladonna** and **Veratrum Viride** are very effectual in relieving congestion of the lungs. **Veratrum Viride** is especially useful here as well as in congestion of the brain.

Hypostatic congestion is a passive congestion occurring simply from weakness after a protracted run of fever or of some affection in which the patient has been obliged to lie in one position a long time, being partly the result of the force of gravity and largely from a weakened heart. **Œdema** of the lungs is a swollen, puffy condition, similar to œdema in other parts. The air cells and tubes are blocked and suffocation results. It is not a primary disease itself, but a complication occurring with diseases of the heart or kidney. **Pulmonary hemorrhage** occurs in two forms: broncho-pulmonary hemorrhage and pulmonary apoplexy. The first form is also called hæmoptysis; in other words, blood spitting.

Hæmoptysis, or blood spitting, may result from different causes, while often a grave symptom, it does not always indicate a serious condition. The points of distinction between hæmorrhage of the lungs and of the stomach are given under the latter heading. Pulmonary apoplexy is the condition where the hemorrhage is into the air cells and interstitial tissue.

Treatment.—In case of hemorrhage of the lungs put the patient to bed and secure absolute physical and mental quiet. A cord may be tied tightly around a limb. Ice may be held in the mouth. Stimulants must not be given. If the patient faints it is nature's way of checking a hemorrhage. We recall a case of frightful hemorrhage that we promptly checked by giving the patient tablespoonsful of Pond's extract or hamamelis, the nearest and only thing we had at hand. Little or no food should be given. Hemorrhages are often produced by errors of diet. The remedies mentioned under nose bleed should be studied. We recall a case of persistent hemorrhage of the lungs which was checked by **Ly-**

copodium. **Aconite, Belladonna** and **Ipecac** are likely to be the indicated remedies. Also study the remedies mentioned under hemorrhage of the stomach.

Pneumonia, sometimes called lung fever, has recently been shown to be an infectious disease of the lungs, caused by a germ named *diplococcus pneumoniæ*. The disease prevails in all climates and is common to all ages. Infants and old persons are especially susceptible to it. In old persons it usually terminates fatally. Debilitated persons generally are more liable to the disease, but none so much so as those addicted to the use of alcoholic liquors. Each attack renders one still more susceptible to another attack.

Symptoms.—The patient may feel indisposed for a day or two or the attack may come on abruptly, with a severe chill, lasting from ten to thirty minutes. The temperature rises quickly and an agonizing pain is felt in the side. A short, dry, painful cough soon develops and the respirations become rapid. By the second or third day the patient lies on the affected side. Cheeks, flushed, the nostrils dilate with hurried breathing, the expression is anxious, the expectorations are tenacious and blood tinged. After seven or nine days the temperature falls within a few hours to normal and the patient as quickly passes from a condition of distress to one of comfort. The crisis may occur sooner or defer to the twelfth or fourteenth day. In severe cases delirium may be present. The disease may affect one or both lungs. The respirations may be as frequent as 40 or 60 or even 80 a minute, that is two, three or four times as rapid as the normal. It is maintained by good old school authorities that pneumonia will run its course uninfluenced by medicines. That it can neither be aborted nor cut short, and furthermore, that under the most unfavorable circumstances, it will often terminate abruptly and naturally without a drop of medicine being given. The death rate from pneumonia under allopathic treatment, according to the same authorities, ranges from 20 to 40 per cent. On the other hand, statistics gathered from many sources, show that the death rate from pneumonia under homeopathic treatment, never reaches 10 per cent. From such conflicting claims we are forced to one of two conclusions. That homeopathic medicine does influence, cut short or abort pneumonia, or that allopathic treatment causes the death of many with this disease, who, if left alone entirely without medicine, would have recovered.

Treatment.—The following homeopathic remedies are those usually indicated in pneumonia: **Aconite, Belladonna, Bryonia, Phosphorus, Tartar Emetic and Veratrum Virdie.** The last is probably the most useful of all in controlling the temperature and pulse. It is well to give this remedy throughout the attack. Poultices are not allowed by many physicians, but after treating cases with and without them we are of the opinion that flaxseed poultices are highly beneficial.

Chronic Interstitial Pneumonia or cirrhosis of the lung is a gradual process by which connective tissue is substituted for the normal tissue of the lung. It is a fibroid change or hardening. It is a chronic disease extending over many years and the patient may enjoy fairly good health; his only annoyance being the cough and shortness of breath. Patients with this disease are generally mistaken for consumptives, but the two affections arise from different causes and are not identical. The cough comes in paroxysms and the expectoration is considerable; indications of dilated or sacculated condition of the bronchi, which has already been described under the term bronchectasis. A fetid odor and hemorrhage occur with a large per cent. of the cases. The affected side of the chest is immobile, retracted and shrunken and presents a striking contrast with the fullness of the sound side. A mild climate and such remedies as the general symptoms indicate is all that can be done in the way of treatment.

Broncho-Pneumonia. or capillary bronchitis, is an inflammation which involves the smallest or terminal branches of the bronchial tubes and the air cells as well, beginning always with the former. Broncho-pneumonia, as a rule, succeeds some infectious disease, as measles, diphtheria, whooping cough, scarlet fever and other fevers. It is a very serious complication in children, causing more deaths than the primary disease. In large cities it ranks in fatality next to infantile diarrhœa. The most common and fatal form of broncho-pneumonia is that which is excited by the bacillus of tuberculosis. In other diseases where there is loss of consciousness and sensibility, particles of food may be drawn into the windpipe and pass down to the smallest branches of the bronchi and develop broncho-pneumonia.

When the patient is under an anæsthetic during a surgical operation about the mouth, foreign particles may be sucked into the lungs and cause the same trouble. Broncho-pneumonia occurs more frequently in children under five years of age. Kicking the clothes off at night and getting chilled accounts, perhaps, for its frequency among them. The death rate, according to old school authorities, ranges from thirty to fifty per cent. Under homeopathic treatment the mortality rate, as far as we can ascertain, is not one-third as great; homeopathic remedies being particularly applicable to this disease in children. **Aconite, Ferrum Phos, Belladonna, Bryonia** and **Chelidonium** should be studied.

Emphysema is that condition in which the air escapes from the lung cells into the spaces between the cells. In post mortem examination the bubbles of air look like rows of beads. The chief symptoms are difficult breathing, lividity, barrel-shaped chest and expiration, requiring more time than inspiration; the reverse of the natural. The condition cannot be corrected. Such subjects are very liable to bronchitis and, therefore, should reside in a mild climate.

Gangrene of the Lung is the result of some other disease in which the blood supply of a part of the lung has been cut off and decay takes place. It may follow the lodgment of a particle of food in a part of the lung or a clot of blood or a plug of the non-absorbable exudate left by pneumonia, or from a pocket of foul mucus in bronchiectasis.

The most striking symptom of gangrene of the lung is the horrible foulness of the expectoration which permeates the atmosphere of the entire room. If the expectoration be allowed to stand in a conical shaped glass it will settle into three distinct layers. At the bottom a greenish brown, heavy sediment; next, a thin liquid of a greenish or brownish tint, and on top a thick, frothy layer. If some of the expectoration be placed upon a piece of glass the shreds of lung tissue may be seen. The fever is moderate and the pulse is rapid. The exhaustion is great and fatal hemorrhage may occur. Recovery may take place. The homeopathic remedies usually indicated are **Arsenicum, Carbo Veg** and **Silicea.**

Abscess of the lung may arise from various causes, but when it follows pnemonia it is easily recognized by the aggravation of the general symptoms by the signs of a cavity and by the character of the expectoration. **Hepar Sulph, Silicea, Phosphorus** and **Sulphur** should be studied.

Pneumonokoniosis embraces those diseases of the lungs due to the inhalation of dust, as coal, iron or stone dust. **New Growths,** or tumors of the lungs, frequently occur after the removal of a cancer from some other part of the body. The development of lung trouble within a year or two after the removal of a cancer indicates recurrence in the lungs.

DISEASES OF THE PLEURA.

As previously stated, the pleura is a shut sac of serous membrane lying between the lung and the ribs. It forms the outer covering of the lung and the inner layer of the chest wall. It may be compared to a flattened bladder without any opening. The diseases of the pleura are as follows: *Acute pleurisy, Chronic pleurisy, Hydrothorax* and *Pneumothorax.* Acute inflammation of the pleura is known as **Acute Pleurisy.** It may come on with a chill and fever, but, as a rule, it develops insidiously, the only noticeable symptom being the distressing pain in the side, usually felt near the nipple or arm pit. It may, however, be felt in the abdomen or low down in the back. The pain is sharp, severe and aggravated by coughing. The fever may rise to 102 or 103, but not so high as in pneumonia. The cough is not so distressing as in pneumonia and it may be absent. The expectoration is usually slight and may be streaked with blood. If much fluid accumulates in the pleural cavity, as it may occur in case of pleurisy, there will be shortness of breath upon exertion, owing to the compression of the lung by the distended pleural sac we have just described. The presence of much fluid may be detected by comparing the two sides of the chest. The affected side will be fuller. The usual depression between the ribs will be absent or pressed out. If the fluid in the pleural sac is pus the condition is called **Empyema**. If the pleural cavity contains only a clear, watery fluid, then the term **Hydrothorax** is applicable to the condition. Should it contain only air, which is a rare condition, we use the term **Pneumothorax**. Should it contain water and air, then the word **Hydropneumothorax** would be applicable, while pyo-pneumothorax would express the combination of pus and air. In case the right pleural cavity is distended the heart will be found pressed over farther to the left side than normal.

Should the distension of the pleural sac reach as high as the collar bone aspiration or tapping is absolutely necessary. It is a simple operation and not attended with much risk or pain, provided it is done by a competent surgeon. When it is determined that there is pus in the pleural sac there should be no hesitation in opening it and treating as an abscess in any other part. Failure to do so costs thousands of lives every year.

Pleurisy, properly treated with such homeopathic remedies as **Apis, Bryonia** and **Arsenicum**, will rarely require tapping. These remedies greatly promote the absorption of fluid in the pleural cavity. If cases have the proper homeopathic treatment from the beginning the unnatural accumulation of fluid in any cavity will be of rare occurrence.

Chronic Pleurisy occurs often as a result of acute pleurisy. Fluid may accumulate and remain for months in the pleural cavity, or it may absorb and the walls of the pleura become stuck together at points, hence the term, pleuritic adhesions. Chronic pleurisy is common in consumption and at times the pain is distressing.

The **Mediastinum**, the space behind the breast-bone and between the lungs, is subject to a number of affections more or less obscure, including tumors, abscesses and inflammation of the lymphatic glands.

SECTION V.

Diseases of the Circulatory System.

DISEASES OF THE PERICARDIUM.

The pericardium is a sac which envelops the heart. **Pericarditis** is inflammation of the pericardium. This condition may arise from direct infection or be secondary to inflammation in some other or neighboring organ. The structure of the pericardium is very similar to the synovial sacs which are found in the larger joints and which is the customary seat of acute articular inflammatory rheumatism. Pericarditis, accompanying or following rheumatism, is a common occurrence. Inflammation of peritoneum, another shut sac, is also frequently followed by inflammation of the pericardium. It may be the sequence less frequently of a number of other diseases, as acute disease of the bone, tuberculosis, scarlet fever or tonsillitis. It may result from extension in pneumonia.

There are three forms of pericarditis. The dry, the moist and the adherent. The first is the most common and usually without pain. It can only be detected by the ear of a skilled physician. The second form is the condition in which water gathers in the pericardial sac and surrounds the heart. This form is often accompanied with considerable pain and distress about the heart. Pressure at the lower end of the breast bone usually aggravates it. There is usually much difficulty in breathing. The patient may be obliged to lie upon the left side or sit up in bed to get his breath. The adherent form include the conditions when there are adhesions. Pericarditis in any form is not necessarily a fatal disease. It is one, however, that is more commonly overlooked than any other. The remedies suggested in case of pleuritis should be studied.

In case of pericarditis arising from inflammatory rheumatism **Cactus, Kalmia** and **Spigelia** should be studied. It is believed that rheumatic pericarditis may be prevented by giving these remedies early, when such a condition is anticipated.

Hydropericardium, called dropsy of the heart, is that condition when the pericardial sac contains fluid. It usually occurs with general dropsy arising from heart or kidney disease. Hæmopericardium is the condition when there is blood in the pericardial sac. When it contains gas it is called pneumo-pericardium. These conditions are rare, but usually fatal within a few hours.

DISEASES OF THE HEART.

Inflammation of the lining membrane of the heart is called **Endocarditis.** The inflammatory process is usually confined to the valves, so that valular endocarditis and endocarditis mean practically the same. It occurs in an acute and a chronic form. The former is distinguished by a tiny vegetation on the valves, generally the result of various infections in other parts of the body. These vegetations undergo changes resulting in thickening of the valves, which may end, in course of time, in organic heart disease. It is in this way that organic heart disease may follow inflammatory rheumatism. Endocarditis is common with pneumonia, also with chorea. As a rule, the patient does not experience any symptoms by which the disease in the simple form can be detected and often the trained ear of a skilled physician hears nothing by which he can make a positive diagnosis.

Chronic Endocarditis, as a rule, results from the acute form and is a slow, insidious process which leads to the deformity of the valves, causing organic heart disease or **Chronic Valvular Disease,** a condition in which the valves are unable to close properly. The inability of the valves to close properly may arise from a change in them or a change in the orifice they guard. Hence, we have the following conditions: Aortic incompetency, aortic stenosis, mitral incompetency, mitral stenosis, tricuspid valve disease, pulmonary valve disease and combined valvular trouble. Persons with great changes in the heart may suffer no inconvenience and live to a good old age, while in other cases an early death may be the result.

Hypertrophy and **Dilatation** of the heart. The former is an enlargement of the heart due to an increase in the thickness of its muscular walls, while dilatation is an enlargement of one or more of its chambers. Hypertrophy of the heart is nature's way of mending some derangement of the valves or arteries. The most common symptom of hypertrophy is a sense of fullness or discomfort about the heart, particularly when the patient lies on the left side.

Myocarditis is an inflammation of the heart muscle. The arteries that supply the heart itself may become diseased and the nutrition of the heart be cut off. In case of protracted fever the nourishment of the heart muscle may be insufficient and it softens just as any other poorly nourished muscle would. The heart muscle may also undergo a **Fatty degeneration,** a condition common in old age and certain diseases. Certain poisons, such as phosphorus, may produce it. **Phosphorus,** homeopathically prepared is, therefore, a remedy for a fatty heart. Sudden deaths are generally the result of some disease of the heart muscle. The first symptoms of such a diseased condition is often a fatal one.

In fleshy persons dizziness, faintness and a feeble pulse do sometimes indicate a fatty heart. In such cases the diet should be studied to reduce the fat in general.

The **Neuroses of the Heart** include palpitation, irregularity of the pulse, rapid pulse, slow pulse and angina pectoris. In perfect health we are unconscious of a heart.

Palpitation is usually a nervous disturbance arising from derangement in some other organ. Dyspepsia, hysteria, tobacco, tea, coffee, loss of sleep and dissipation generally, may produce it. Orificial surgery, the correction of any derangement of the lower orifices, will generally steady the heart. The condition in which the pulse now and then skips a beat is often corrected by **Digitalis** or **Gelsemium.** Soon after child birth a woman's pulse may be as low as 44 and be natural. A slow pulse is common in those who have had rheumatism, pneumonia, typhoid and diphtheria. Hunger and digestive troubles may produce a slow pulse. **Angina Pectoris,** a rare disease, comes on with violent paroxysms of pain in the heart, extending to the arms and neck, with a sensation of dying. **Glonoin** is the indicated remedy.

False angina pectoris is common and is due to some nervous disturbance and may call for different remedies.

For affections of the heart in general the following remedies should be studied: **Digitalis, Gelsemium, Arsenicum, Rhus Tox, Spigelia, Cactus, Kalmia, Veratrum Alb., Lachesis, Cimicifuga** and **Glonoin.** While arsenicum is not supposed to have any special action upon the heart we have seen a rapid, feeble pulse change to one stronger, steadier and twenty beats slower within ten minutes after giving a dose of that remedy; given not for the heart alone, but because the general symptoms of the patient presented a picture of that remedy; another beautiful illustration of the wonderful and accurate adaptability of the homeopathic law.

DISEASES OF THE ARTERIES.

Longevity depends very much upon the condition of the arteries. It is said that a "man is only as old as his arteries." The arteries may undergo fatty degeneration, calcification, sclerosis or hardening. The latter condition is generally produced by alcohol, lead, gout, syphilis, over-eating and over-drinking. **Aneurism** is the condition when at some point in its course an artery becomes greatly distended from weakness of its walls. Cases of aneurism have been reported cured by **Lycopodium.** Valvular troubles have also been improved by its use.

SECTION VI.

Diseases of the Blood.

ANÆMIA.

The reduction of the amount of the blood as a whole or of its corpuscles or of some of its other elements, such as albumen or hæmoglobin, is termed Anæmia. This condition may be from different causes. A hemorrhage produces anæmia in proportion to its amount. The total amount of blood in an average sized adult is about ten pounds. The sudden loss of three or four pounds of blood may produce death. Anæmia may be produced by the long continued loss of albumen in Bright's disease and other exhausting diseases. It may also be produced by defective nourishment. Poisonous drugs will produce anæmia, such as lead, mercury and arsenic. The virus of syphilis and malaria are very destructive to the red corpuscles. Hence, anæmia is common in this disease. **Chlorosis** is a form of anæmia very common among girls between the ages of fourteen and seventeen, who are ill-fed, overworked, closely confined in badly lighted and ventilated rooms and who have a great deal of stair climbing to do. Cases may occur under the most favorable conditions. Mental and emotional disturbances, no doubt, often cause it. It has followed disappointment in love affairs. Good blood contains about five million blood corpuscles to a cubic millimeter. In all cases of chlorosis the number is considerably less. But the greatest change is in the amount of hæmoglobin, the iron containing element of the blood; it may fall below fifty per cent. of the normal. The amount of iron in the blood is also less. Girls with chlorosis do not lose in weight. Their complexion is of a peculiar yellow green, from which fact it is sometimes called green sickness. The lips, gums and tongue are deathly pale. They get out of breath upon the slightest exertion and have palpitation of the heart. Faint, easily. The appetite is changeable, but there is generally a craving for something sour. In some cases they will eat all sorts of things, as chalk, slate pencils, or even earth. Menstrual disturbances are common in such cases. Constipation is obstinate. **Sulphur, Pulsatilla, Ferrum** and **Arsenicum,** along with electricity, will cure most cases of chlorosis. We have seen remarkable improvement in such cases follow orificial surgery. There is a severe form of anæmia called **Pernicious Anæmia,** in which the number of red corpuscles is reduced to one-tenth of the normal, while the hæmoglobin is relatively increased; the opposite of chlorosis. The skin has a smooth, waxy, blanched appearance. The lips, gums and tongue are bloodless. There is extreme languor and faintness, yet, after months of this trouble, the body remains as plump as usual. **Arsenicum** and **Apis** are usually indicated.

Leukæmia is that condition of the blood in which there is a persistent increase of the white blood corpuscles associated with enlargement of the spleen, or of the lymphatic glands, or of the marrow of the bones. The average number of white corpuscles to a cubic millimeter of healthy blood is about 6,000, while that of the red is about 5,000,000; the normal ratio between the two is about 1 to 800. In leukæmia the white may increase so that this ratio may be 1 to 10 or even 1 to 1. Like anæmia it comes on insidiously and the general appearance may resemble that disease. But the patient generally consults a physician first for the enlarged abdomen and shortness of breath, or for enlarged glands. The disease usually terminates fatally within two or three years. **Arsenicum** is usually the indicated remedy, although other remedies should be studied.

Hodgkin's Disease begins with enlargement of the glands of the neck, of the arm pits and of the groin, along with anæmia. It differs from tubercular enlargement of the glands in that the glands are uniformly enlarged on both sides of the body. The lymphatic glands about the bronchi may enlarge and cause suffocation. Acute cases may terminate fatally within three or four months, while the chronic may live as many years. **Phosphorus** should be studied for this disease, also **Iodine** and **Arsenicum.**

Addison's Disease, in the language of the man whose name it bears, is described as follows: "Anæmia, general languor or debility, remarkable feebleness of heart's action, irritability of the stomach and a peculiar change of the color of the skin." The pigmentation of the skin is usually the first symptom that attracts attention. The color of which may vary from a light yellow to a deep brown or even black. The disease is supposed to originate in the nervous system of the abdomen, especially that part which supplies the kidneys. There are a number of other conditions in which pigmentation of the skin occur. But the great weakness of Addison's disease will distinguish it. The disease is usually fatal.

The term **Blood Poisoning** is commonly applied to septicæmia, but the blood contains poison in case of syphilis, malaria and many other diseases.

DISEASES OF THE THYROID GLAND.

Goitre is an enlargement of the thyroid gland and gives a swollen appearance of the sides of the front part of the neck. It is more common in some countries than in others. It is very common in the mountainous countries of Switzerland. Goitre may become so large as to interfere with breathing. **Spongia, Calcarea Carb** and **Iodine** are the chief homeopathic remedies. Electricity is generally effective in reducing goitre.

The following tumors may occur in the thyroid gland: Adenomata, cancer and sarcoma.

Exopthalmic Goitre, sometimes called Graves's disease, also Basedow's disease, is a goitre accompanied by a bulging out of the eye balls, giving an ox-like look about the eyes. Worry, fright and depressing emotions usually precede the disease. Disturbances of the heart usually precede and accompany the disease. It may disappear in the course of a few months or continue for years.

Myxœdema is known by an edematous or swollen condition of the skin about the thyroid gland and adjacent parts. The swelling is inelastic and does not pit on pressure, as in case of true edema. It tends to obliterate and distort the expression of the face; giving an idiotic or imbecile look, which represents the true condition of the mind. The thyroid gland degenerates or shrinks.

The disease occurs five times more frequently among women than among men. It is a slow, but progressive disease and may extend over a period of ten or fifteen years. The disease is very peculiar and is not likely to be mistaken for any other disease, except Bright's. But the absence of albumen in the urine and the absence of pitting on pressure readily distinguishes it from that disease. Such patients suffer greatly from cold. A warm climate is recommended.

SECTION VII.

Diseases of the Kidneys.

Most of the information concerning the condition of the kidneys is obtained by a chemical and microscopical examination of the urine. A diseased condition of the kidney may thus be discovered long before there are any other symptoms by which it could be detected by the patient or the physician. A healthy adult should pass on the average three pints of water within twenty-four hours. The passing of a much larger or smaller quantity than this amount for any considerable time indicates something abnormal; an excessive amount usually indicating diabetes.

A decrease of the amount of urine is met in acute fevers. Profuse sweating will decrease the quantity of urine, while a sudden change of weather from warm to cold will increase it. The drinking of a large quantity of beer or certain kinds of mineral waters will also increase the quantity. The specific gravity of normal urine is not, as a rule, below 1015 nor above 1025; the average being

1020. If it remains long outside of these limits there is a diseased condition somewhere. If above 1025 it suggests diabetes mellitus, or acute Bright's disease. If below 1015 diabetes insipidus or chronic Bright's disease of the interstitial variety. Sugar in the urine indicates diabetes mellitus, while albumen points to Bright's disease. Pus in the urine suggests an abscess of the kidney, while blood in small quantities would lead us to suspect renal calculi or gravel of the kidney. An excess of uric acid indicates disturbances of nutrition. Alkaline urine, bladder trouble.

Movable Kidney or floating kidney is sometimes met. It rarely causes any disturbance. **Congestion of the Kidneys** of an acute nature may be caused by cold, poisons and such irritants, as turpentine, cubebs, cantharides or copaiba. There is an intimate relation between the kidneys and the skin. Chilling of the skin quickly affects the kidneys. The continued absence of sweat is one of the most common symptoms of Bright's disease. Passive congestion of the kidneys may occur in chronic disease of the heart and lungs, also by pressure in pregnancy and dropsy.

Hæmaturia or blood in the urine may accompany a number of diseases or it may be produced by irritating drugs. A common cause is gravel in the kidney or bladder. It may also come from a fall or a blow on the back over the region of the kidney. Blood in the urine gives it a red, smoky color. If the blood comes from the bladder it is present only in the last part of the water passed. If the blood comes from the kidney it will be uniformly mixed with the urine. Whether the blood in the urine comes from the kidney or the bladder may be determined by washing out the bladder. In case it is from the bladder the water will be blood-tinged, but if it is from the kidney the water will be clear. Rest in bed and a milk diet is the best treatment for hæmaturia. **Belladonna, Phosphorus** or **Hamamelis** may be indicated.

The term, **Albuminuria,** indicates the condition when albumen is present in the urine. The white of an egg is an example of pure albumen. If it be put into pure water and boiled it will be precipitated into a white mass. Likewise the presence of albumen in urine is tested by boiling. If no cloudiness or precipitate occurs it is a positive sign that there is no albumen. If the urine becomes cloudy on boiling it indicates either the presence of albumen or phosphates. The addition of nitric acid will cause the phosphates to dissolve and clear up the water, but if the cloudiness is due to albumen it will become only more cloudy upon the addition of nitric acid.

Not every person who has albumen in the urine has Bright's disease, but, as a rule, every person with Bright's disease has albumen in the urine. Albuminuria may arise from eating food very rich in albumen, violent muscular exertion, violent emotions, cold bathing and dyspepsia, as well as from organic disease of the kidney, such as Bright's. Albumen in small quantities may occur in young unmarried persons of both sexes. White of egg, lean meat and cheese are some of the best samples of albuminous food. The quantity of albumen in the urine may be increased or diminished at will by a change of diet. A diet containing the least amount of albumen will be attended with the least albumen in the urine. Albumen is generally present in the urine of all cases of severe infectious diseases, such as diphtheria, scarlet fever and pneumonia. Life insurance companies reject all applicants for insurance who have albumen in the urine.

Pyuria is the term used to express pus in the urine. In large abscesses of the kidney the pus may appear only intermittently, while in cases of pus developed from a stone or from tuberculosis of the kidney the pus appears constantly. In case the pus is due to cystitis, that is, inflammation of the bladder, it will be ropy and the urine alkaline and foul. The pus of urethritis, particularly that of gonorrhœa, will appear with the first water passed and there will be local evidences of inflammation of the urethra. If the pus is due to the escape of some neighboring abscess into the urinary passage a considerable quantity will come at one time and then it will cease. There will also be other symptoms that such an abscess has formed. Urine containing pus has a white or yellowish white appearance. A heavy grayish sediment is seen on settling and the fluid above it is turbid. The sediment is sometimes ropy and tough. Urine containing pus is generally alkaline and has a peculiar, foul, stale odor, called ammoniacal. Pus corpuscles may be seen under the microscope.

Lithuria, uric acid in the urine, has been discussed elsewhere under the heading, Lithæmia. The amount of uric acid in the urine depends upon the diet. It is least with a vegetable diet and greatest with an animal diet. Fifteen grains of salicylate of sodium, given three times a day, will greatly increase the amount of uric acid in the urine for two days. At the beginning of typhoid fever and a number of other complaints the patient usually suffers a great deal of pain here and there, which is commonly called rheumatic. We have repeatedly observed the fact that salicylate of sodium given for twenty-four hours, five grains every four hours, will relieve the pain as if by magic, but have no other or further influence upon the course of the disease. This leads us to the conclusion that such pains are due to an excess of uric acid in the blood and the salicylate of sodium simply removes the excess of acid. **Oxaluria** is a combination of oxalic acid and lime that is sometimes found in the urine. A diet of tomatoes, rheubarb and the like increases it. It is associated with dyspeptic disturbances and is included in the term lithæmia.

Phosphaturia is a combination of phosphoric acid and some mineral elements, as potassium, sodium, calcium and magnesium. With lime and magnesia it forms the earthy phosphates, which are sometimes found in the bladder and are passed with the last portion of the urine, giving it a cloudy, milky appearance. This condition has been mistaken for spermatorrhœa. In severe, wasting diseases, as phthisis, anæmia and the like, the phosphates are increased in the urine, but decreased in acute diseases.

Indicanuria is the name given to the condition when the urine contains indigo. It is met in peritonitis, empyema and obstinate constipation. A milk diet increases it. To test for indican boil a quantity of nitric acid and to it add an equal quantity of urine. A bluish ring develops at the point of contact. Now add a quantity of chloroform equal to the quantity of acid and urine combined. Shake and on standing the chloroform will have a violet or bluish color, due to the presence of indigo in the urine.

Uræmia is due to retention in the blood of poisonous elements that should be excreted with the urine. It is usually associated with inflammation of the kidneys or Bright's disease, but pressure upon the kidneys may produce it or it may occur in cases where the blood is greatly changed, as in case of cholera. Uræmia may be manifested by brain, lung or bowel symptoms. Uræmia may come on suddenly in persons who have had no previous mental disturbances and who were not supposed to have Bright's disease.

Delusional insanity may occur, followed by suicide. Convulsions may develop suddenly and unexpectedly. Profound unconsciousness may come on. Various forms of palsies may result. Headache in the back part of the head and neck is common. Difficult breathing may come on in paroxysms or it may be continuous. But usually there are attacks of difficult breathing at night, resembling true asthma. The patient must sit up and gasp for breath. There may be nausea and severe vomiting. Or, the bowels may be very loose. The tongue and breath are usually very foul.

Treatment.—In case of convulsions from uræmia or from any other cause strip and wrap the patient with sheets wrung out of hot water. Inject into the bowel two or three quarts of warm water. In case of profound unconsciousness arising from uræmia pursue the same course. The homeopathic preparation of **Turpentine** 3x, may also be given internally. The headache and fullness of the head occurring from uræmia will be relieved by **Glonoin**, 3x. The asthmatic attacks will be best relieved by drop doses of **Digitalis** tincture. The nausea, vomiting and diarrhœa caused by uræmia is best met by **Arsenicum** 3x. The diarrhœa, however, seems to be nature's way of getting rid of the poison which the kidneys cannot eliminate.

Acute Bright's Disease, or acute diffuse nephritis, is an acute inflammation of the kidneys and may arise from cold, from the poisons of infectious fevers, particularly scarlet fever, from poisonous drugs, as turpentine, cantharides, carbolic acid and the like, from pregnancy and from extensive burns or injury to the skin. Acute Bright's disease from cold comes on suddenly. A puffy condition of the face and ankles may be noticed within twenty-four hours. But after fevers it is slower in developing. There may be nausea, vomiting, chilliness, pain in the back and fever. The urine may be suppressed at first or it may be scanty, highly colored and contain albumen, blood and tube casts. Only four or five ounces may be passed within twenty-four hours. The specific gravity will be 1025 or higher. Serious disease of the kidneys may exist with no other symptoms than a slight puffiness about the eyes and ankles. Acute Bright's disease very frequently develops during the third week of scarlet fever and causes many deaths. Every case of scarlet fever should be carefully watched and guarded until after the third week.

Treatment.—Recovery is the rule in case of acute Bright's disease, while the opposite is the usual result of the chronic. The patient should be put to bed and kept warm by blankets. The diet should be milk or non-albuminous food, such as gruels made of arrow root, oat meal or barley. An exclusive milk diet is usually the best. No meat or eggs should be allowed. **Arsenicum, Apis, Belladonna, Rhus Tox, Turpentine** and **Sulphur** may be indicated.

Chronic Bright's Disease occurs in two forms: *Chronic Parenchymatous Nephritis* and *Chronic Interstitial Nephritis.* The former is attended with considerable dropsy, while in the latter dropsy is either absent or comes on late. The following terms are also used to express the first form: *Chronic Desquamative Nephritis, Chronic Tubal Nephritis* and *Chronic Diffuse Nephritis with Exudation.* To the second form is applied the terms: *Contracted Kidney, Granular Kidney, Cirrhosis of the Kidney, Gouty Kidney* and *Renal Sclerosis.* The first form, **Chronic Parenchymatous Nephritis,** may follow the acute or it may come on insidiously from a number of other causes, among which may be mentioned: Alcohol, beer, chronic suppuration, syphilis and tuberculosis. The chronic may come on very much like the acute, or there may be dyspepsia, failing of strength and puffiness in the morning of the eyelids and ankles. The urine is scanty, smoky or a dirty yellow. Albumen is abundant, amounting to one-third or one-half of the volume of the urine boiled. But the positive symptom of the disease is ascertained only by the microscope, namely, the presence of hyaline, granular or fatty tube casts. Dropsy comes on early in this form and is persistent. Uræmic symptoms are common. The heart and eyes are less affected in this than in the second form; we refer to chronic interstitial nephritis. The specific gravity of the urine is usually too low in the latter stages of chronic Bright's disease, the opposite of the condition in the acute. The outlook for a case of this kind of Bright's disease, which has lasted for a year, is not encouraging.

Treatment.—A milk diet is best. Albuminous food should be avoided, of which eggs, lean meat and cheese are the best examples. **Apis, Arsenicum, Phosphorus, Turpentine, Rhus Tox, Sulphur** and many other remedies may be beneficial. Mineral waters containing much iron has been highly beneficial in some cases. The circulation may be improved and the dropsy lessened by orificial surgery.

Chronic Interstitial Nephritis is known under several different names, which we have just enumerated above and which are more or less descriptive of the condition of the kidneys during this form of Bright's disease. It may result from the form we have just described or it may develop independently or it may be produced by a hardened condition of the arteries. The tendency to the disease may be inherited. Errors of diet, an excessive use of meat and alcoholic liquors are important factors in causing the disease. Along with over-eating and over-drinking must be mentioned hurried eating, worry and mental strain from great business cares. This form is frequently met in men prominent in business or political circles. It was this form of Bright's that caused the death of the Hon. James G. Blaine. It rarely occurs in persons under forty years of age. The majority of cases are not discovered until well advanced. It is thought that the disease may remain latent for a long time until some other disease suddenly starts it up. A case in point occurs to us. A man forty-five years old, of sedentary habits, a hearty eater and a great mental worker, was seized with the grip during holidays. He was confined to bed a few days, but soon returned to his office and began work again as usual. He noticed, however, that he passed a larger quantity of urine than natural and had it examined. Albumen was found in abundance; also fatty and granular tube casts. But a close examination revealed that he had had nausea mornings for months and that for the same length of time he had been obliged to rise several times a night to urinate. His eye-sight had been failing for some time. Asthmatic attacks had troubled him occasionally for some time, attended with pain in the heart. Climbing stairs took his breath. The specific gravity of his urine was 1010 and the amount was fully six pints, but when dropsy set in, a month before his death, it diminished to a pint. He became nearly blind. The distressing attacks of difficult breathing was of daily occurrence. He frequently vomited. Matzoon, a milk preparation similar to koumiss, was the only article of food that agreed with him throughout his sickness. **Digitalis** in the tincture relieved the heart attacks; **Glonoin**, the headache and fullness; **Apis**, the rolling of the head; **Arsenicum**, the intense thirst and deathly look; **Rhus Tox**, the backache, and **Lycopodium**, the coated tongue. While the end was fatal four months after the attack of the grip, treatment, we are sure, prolonged his life and made his last days as easy as possible. In this way, also, homeopathic treatment may be said to be successful even though the patient dies.

Amyloid, waxy or lardaceous degeneration of the kidney is only a stage in chronic Bright's disease, usually met in those cases following fevers, syphilis, tuberculosis or prolonged suppuration, and which show evidence of enlargement of the spleen or liver. During this stage a large quantity of pale urine of low specific gravity is passed and it may contain pus.

Pyelitis includes Consectutive nephritis, Pyelonephritis and Pyonephrosis. It is an inflammation of the lining of the pelvis or cavity of the kidney. It may arise from the irritation of gravel, tubercle, infectious diseases, foul urine, cancer or tumor. Excepting gravel, the most common cause is extension of inflammation in the bladder to the kidney. When such is the case the body of the kidney usually becomes involved and the result is the surgical kidney or acute suppurative nephritis. Pyelitis, associated with fevers, usually comes on during convalescence and may have no positive symptoms. The urine is cloudy and acid. Pain and tenderness in the back are usually present. In case of suppurative pyelitis there are chills and fever, which may be intermittent or assume a typhoid character. There may be or there may not be pain in the back. To detect this condition early is important, as it may be the means of saving the patient's life by resorting to a surgical operation for relieving the pus. We recall a case of this kind in which, if we had known as much a week before as we did after the post mortem examination, we might have saved the man's life by operating and removing the pint of pus in the kidney before it poisoned him to death. In this case we could not discover any pain or tenderness over the kidney, but a great deal in the bladder. He had had catarrh of the bladder for a year. The urine was horribly foul and contained blood and pus. Fever was present two weeks before death and it resembled typhoid so much that one of the consulting physicians was inclined to think it nothing else.

Hydronephrosis is a dilatation of the cavity of the kidney from an accumulation of water. It may be congenital or acquired. It may be mistaken for a tumor. The sac may be tapped and the fluid drawn off.

Nephrolithiasis, or renal calculus, develops by the solid constituents of the urine, forming concretions or gravel. The concretions may form out of a number of substances and may vary in size from a pea to a hickory nut and even much larger. They may form in great numbers. Some escaping with the urine and others remaining for years, causing much or little disturbance. The passing of a large gravel may be attended with the most intense pain, which may be mistaken for biliary colic or intestinal colic. But in renal colic the pain will extend from the kidney to the bladder, in the line of the ureter through which it travels from the kidney to the bladder. As soon as the stone reaches the bladder the intense pain ceases. This fact alone is sufficient to determine the nature of the trouble. An ancient writer describes the passing of renal calculus as follows: "Thou art seen to sweat with pain, to look pale and red, to tremble, to vomit well nigh to blood, to suffer strange contortions and convulsions, by starts to let tears drop from thine eyes, to urine thick, black, frightful water or to have it suppressed

by some sharp and craggy stone that cruelly pricks and tears thee."
The urine is passed frequently and usually contains blood.

Treatment.— A hot bath usually gives the most relief. It may be necessary to resort to chloroform or morphine. Hot cloths or poultices, applied over the region of the pain, may give relief. Persons suffering from gravel should drink daily a large quantity of distilled water, to which has been added the citrate or bicarbonate of potash. Large stones are now successfully and safely removed by a surgical operation; opening up the kidney. The diet should be vegetable. **Lycopodium** is often indicated.

Tumors of the Kidneys may be either benign or malignant. Clotted blood or bloody casts in the urine points to cancer of the kidney. The symptoms of **Cystic** disease of the kidney resembles those of chronic interstitial nephritis and during life the disease cannot be positively determined. **Perinephric abscess**, that is an abscess in the tissues about the kidney may occur from an injury or from an extension of a suppurative process in some neighboring part, the kidney, the appendix or the bowel. Such abscesses come on slowly. There is pain in the lumbar region, aggravated by pressure and extending down into the hip and inner side of the thigh. The testicle on the affected side is usually retracted. Puffiness of the skin is frequently present. In children the disease has been mistaken for disease of the hip joint. The **Treatment** is to open the abscess and drain out the pus, thoroughly.

DISEASES OF THE BLADDER.

Diseases of the **Urethra** must be included with those of the bladder, since it is to the bladder what the spout is to the tea-kettle.

The average capacity of the bladder is eight ounces, but it may be so contracted as to contain only a few drachms, or it may be so dilated as to hold a gallon. The bladder may be absent, it may be too large or too small, it may be baggy, or sacculated. Besides gravel there has been found in the bladder pins, needles, pieces of straw, glass tubing, pipe stems, lead pencils and many other **foreign bodies**, inserted at the suggestion of budding sexual instincts. Various injuries of the bladder may occur. **Rupture** of the bladder is generally due to a fall or a crushing. It is indicated by severe pain and a fruitless desire to urinate. Collapse or a fatal peritonitis usually follows. The treatment is to open the bladder, wash out and sew up the rent. **Perforating ulcer** of the bladder may occur. **Atony** of the bladder is due to a weakness of the muscular wall and is indicated by a corresponding loss of power in expressing the water from the bladder. Every male past middle life notices that he cannot eject as forcible a stream as in boyhood. Atony may come on gradually and even naturally, but it may develop suddenly from active disease of the bladder.

Retention of the Urine is a natural consequence of atony. In retention the bladder fills up with urine, but it cannot be passed. Retention should not be confounded with **Suppression of Urine.** The latter is that condition in which no urine is secreted and none is found in the bladder. Retention may be readily detected by examining the abdomen over the region of the bladder. Besides atony, retention may be caused by an enlarged prostate tumor or stricture of the urethra. Voluntary retention may lead to involuntary retention. In certain febrile diseases or after childbirth the bladder may be so benumbed that retention passes unnoticed by the patient. There may be partial retention, indicated by frequent micturition and dribbling of urine. The urine retained is termed residual. If this amount is four ounces the catheter should be used every twelve hours. If it amounts to eight ounces then the catheter should be used every eight hours. Electricity is beneficial in stimulating the weakened muscles. **Gelsemium, Nux Vomica, Belladonna, Cantharis, Conium, Pulsatilla** and many other remedies may be more or less useful. **Incontinence of Urine,** or bed-wetting is common among children. The term nocturnal enuresis is frequently applied to this condition. **Belladonna** or **Pulsatilla,** along with moral suasion, is usually all that is necessary in such cases. A long foreskin, however, is often the cause of incontinence of urine in boys, not only at night, but in the day time. Circumcision is the remedy. Incontinence or dribbling of the urine in case of adults usually indicates retention.

Vesical tenesmus is a straining to urinate, usually more or less continuous, and aggravated after some water has been passed. It occurs with a number of diseases or fevers. Hæmaturia, or bloody urine, has been discussed in connection with diseases of the kidneys. The blood may come from the kidney, the bladder or the urethra. If the blood is from the fore part of the urethra some of it will escape between urinations. Blood from the kidney is usually accompanied with a pain or heaviness in the small of the back. **Neuralgia of the Bladder** is indicated by frequent desire to pass water. When once asleep or pleasantly occupied the desire is less frequent, but on damp, rainy days, or when worried, the desire is more frequent. The spirits are usually depressed. It is distinguished from cystitis, which is also accompanied by frequent micturition, by the fact that in the former the urine is free from pus, while in the latter it is not. We have just dismissed, as cured, a case of neuralgia of the neck of the bladder, which was an exceedingly aggravated one. The despondency was very great, amounting to an attempt of suicide. The treatment consisted in dilating the urethra and the rectum to the limit. Some papillae and hemorrhoids were removed from the rectum. Within two months the patient, who had been sick a year, was transformed from a pale, bloodless, nervous, suspicious, despondent person, to a most jolly and rosy cheeked young lady.

Acute Cystitis is inflammation of the bladder. It is usually confined to the mucous coat or inner layer of the bladder, although the deeper layers and even the peritoneal coat covering the bladder may be involved. Acute cystitis may arise from five different causes: Injury or mechanical irritation, extension of inflammation from urethra, aggravation of a chronic inflammation, drugs and nervous troubles. Whatever the cause, the symptoms are much the same. The calls to urinate are frequent and imperative night and day. Micturition is not followed by relief. There is smarting pain and tenesmus. Heavy burning pain is felt between the legs beneath the bladder, and over the bladder, radiating down the thigh to the end of the penis and up into the loins. The urine contains pus which is often passed in strings of mucus. Hence, the name catarrh of the bladder. The urine is acid at first, but becomes alkaline. The fever may run high and there may be a dry tongue, restlessness and even hiccough in case of gangrene.

Chronic Catarrh or cystitis is the most frequent of all diseases of the bladder. It is always the result of some other disease, as a stone in the bladder or kidney, obstruction of the urethra, neuralgia of the neck of the bladder, excessive acid urine, diseases of the kidney. The symptoms of chronic cystitis resemble those of the acute, into which any time it may suddenly develop. The urine is always cloudy and contains pus. The pus may not be seen by the naked eye or it may be precipitated into clots or ropes, if the urine becomes or is made alkaline. To determine the presence of pus in urine add ammonia. Its presence will then be quite apparent. Chronic cystitis is most successfully treated by removing its cause. If a stricture is the cause dilate with steel rounds. If a stone in the kidney or bladder, remove it. If due to foul urine, wash out the bladder regularly.

The awful tenesmus that sometimes occurs in cystitis is relieved by ten drop doses of the tincture of **Hyoscyamus**. A tea of triticum repens or couch grass gives great relief and is, in some cases of cystitis, all that is necessary.

The chief symptoms of **Stone in the Bladder** are as follows: Desire to urinate more frequent during the day than at night. Darting, burning pains felt during micturition, but more severe immediately after. The pain is generally felt on the under surface of the penis near the end. During urination sudden interruption of the stream, due to the blocking of the passage by the stone. Blood, pus and pains in various parts are only confirmatory symptoms. As just observed in regard to the location of the pain in case of stone in the bladder, it is well to remember that in other diseases of the genito-urinary organs the pain is not always at the seat of difficulty. For instance, in case of kidney disease the pain is usually in the groin, the testicle or down the thigh, while in disease of the testicle the pain is in the groin. The benefit to the whole nervous system derived from dilating the urethra in case of an irritable bladder by means of **steel sounds** is very great. The most common of all genito-urinary troubles is inflammation of the urethra, called **Urethritis**, and attended with more or less discharge. There are two forms; the one simple and the other specific. To the latter the term, **Gonorrhœa** or clap, has been given. Though a companion to syphilis it is an entirely different disease. The only resemblance between them being the fact that both usually involve the sexual organs and both are usually associated with sexual immorality.

It is impossible, without the microscope, to determine to which form of urethritis some cases belong.

A healthy young husband may acquire from his equally healthy young wife or vice versa, a severe urethritis, attended with abundant discharge which may appear to be exactly like that of gonorrhœa. In the discharge of simple urethritis only pus microbes will be found, while in that of specific urethritis or gonorrhœa, a germ known as **gonococcus** will be present. Gonorrhœa in those infected for the first time begins as follows: A period after exposure varying from a few hours to two weeks, but usually within a week, the patient notices a milk-and-water-like fluid at the mouth of the urethra which is reddened and swollen. A tickling or scalding sensation is soon felt, especially after urinating. Within forty-eight hours these symptoms are all greatly aggravated. The passing of the urine is attended with the most acute suffering. Tenesmus is also severe. The discharge at first like diluted milk becomes white and thicker and then yellow and then greenish, streaked with blood. After four or five days the symptoms become less severe, but may continue for weeks, the discharge growing less all the time. However, a chronic urethritis called **gleet** may follow and persist for months and even years. A painful swelling may occur in the groin. The testicle may swell and be very painful. This is especially liable to happen if powerful astringent injections are used to suppress the discharge. A very common complication is when the inflammation extends to the bladder and develops cystitis. It will be remembered that the inflammation of cystitis may extend, in course of time, to the kidney and suppurative pyelitis or abscess of the kidney result. Thus, instead of being a temporary matter of little consequence gonorrhœa is often attended with serious and long lasting complication which may result in death. Under homeopathic treatment such complications are less likely to occur and if they have already been established from violent measures, homeopathic remedies will undo the mischief in the most satisfactory manner. During the acute stage no injections should be used unless it is pure water or a weak solution of peroxide of hydrogen, for the sake of cleanliness. Bathing the penis in a cup of hot water will relieve the severe pain. The homeopathic remedy during this stage is **Aconite**, 2x, given every hour. Later, **Belladonna, Gelsemium** and **Mercurius** may be needed. For complications, **Sulphur, Gelsemium, Bryonia, Pulsatilla, Hepar Sulph.** and **Sepia** may be indicated. Complications from suppressing the discharge of gonorrhœa have existed for years and the discharge has been re-established by a dose of **Sepia**; the case then running a regular course, as if it were a recent or fresh infection.

Stricture of the urethra is another complication usually following gonorrhœa. It is the result of the inflamed walls during urethritis, becoming united in places and narrowing the canal of the urethra so much in some cases that the water can hardly pass. Even complete obstruction may occur, or the urine containing pus may burrow a new canal for its escape. Such a canal is termed a **urinary fistula** and usually opens somewhere on the under side of the penis. In case of complete obstruction it is sometimes necessary to tap the bladder through the abdominal wall.

SECTION VIII.

Diseases of the Sexual System.

SEXUAL ABUSE.

A complete description of the diseases of the sexual organs and an enumeration of the perversions of the sexual instincts would fill volumes. Excepting self preservation, the perpetuation of the species is the strongest human instinct. The sexual instinct manifests itself at an early age and is very liable to be perverted. The habit of self-abuse or masturbation may be formed in boys as early as the fifth year, although usually not until the twelfth or fourteenth year. We have known girls to begin as early as the tenth year. The habit is very common among boys, and is supposed to be less common among girls. But during the past year more cases of girls than of boys have come under our professional care. The damage done to the nervous system was fully as great as in cases of boys.

The evil effects of the habit cannot be overdrawn. It takes away the elasticity of the body and the vivacity of the mind. In place it leaves a listless, stupid indifference, with pale, sunken cheeks and hollow eyes. In girls it destroys that indefinable sweetness which is their natural attraction. To one of the opposite sex in a normal condition they are offensive. It is not unusual for the face of those who practice the habit to become pimply. Yet a pimply face does not always indicate the habit. A few years ago a young woman of twenty-two came under our care for a horribly pimply face. She was a devoted Christian, engaged in active charity work. She was also wealthy and for four years had traveled far and near, spending money lavishly to have her face cured. During all this time she had never had a beau. After treating her several weeks and having exhausted all our medical resources in vain upon her case, we resolved to tell her, at any cost, our first impression of her case, namely, that she was indulging in a secret habit that was ruining her health and was the prime cause of her pimply face. Imagine our embarrassment, when she positively denied, in the most truthful manner, our accusation, and almost led us to believe that a sexual thought had never entered her mind. Again, imagine our surprise when, two days later, she confessed of having indulged in the habit perhaps four hundred times in four years. Never until we accused her did she have the remotest idea that the habit was affecting her health or was at all sinful. She reproached her mother because she had not been instructed and warned against the evil habit. She at once gave up the habit. Our remedies took effect. Within two months afterwards her face was perfectly smooth and she looked five hundred per cent. more attractive. Another young woman confessed that at the age of ten years she indulged for a time in the habit. Since then she has positively loathed everything sexual and has refused good offers of marriage because of her unnatural repugnance to sexual matters. Though indulged in at such an early age she bears upon her face as well as in her mind the unmistakable imprint of the habit. Besides causing mental and physical debility amounting to dementia and even epilepsy, self abuse leaves a weakness that remains long after the habit has been overcome. This weakness consists in seminal losses upon the slightest provocation, followed by a sense of mental and physical exhaustion.

These losses, called **Spermatorrhœa**, usually occur during sleep, being provoked by lustful dreams. Females who have practiced self abuse suffer sometimes in later years in a similar manner. In consequence of which the nervous system is affected seriously. After marriage a premature loss of semen is a common complaint of those who have practiced self abuse during boyhood. This, to a wife in a normal condition, is decidedly disagreeable and has more than once led to divorce or something worse. Total impotency on the part of the male and total indifference on the part of the female may result from self abuse. A towel wrung out of cold, salt watei and applied to the privates on retiring is the simplest treatment for spermatorrhœa. Steel sounds passed into the bladder are also highly beneficial. Great good is derived from the steady and persistent use of electricity. A fruit and vegetable diet lessens the tendency to seminal losses, while a stimulating diet, including meat, tea, coffee, liquors, peppers and sauces tend to aggravate the trouble. Regular and systematic exercise, not over-exertion, is beneficial. It is needless to say that everything suggesting lewd thoughts must be banished from the mind. The society of a company of refined ladies and gentlemen is of a great advantage. A number of homeopathic remedies are of service among which are **Nux Vom., Belladonna, Arsenicum, Gelsemium** and **Calcarea Carb.** The rectum should be examined and all irritation there removed,

Rectal trouble, especially constipation, is very common in masturbators. A blunting of the sexual instinct is often occasioned by too frequent indulgence and may lead to repugnance for each other in a couple who had been mutually attractive. Indulgence more than once a week is rarely compatible with the highest degree of health and pleasure. Many a domestic quarrel and divorce proceeding begin with the repugnance mentioned above. A temporary separation is the remedy. Let the one most at fault visit for a few weeks another climate. Perfect health and perfect love are the essential factors for the highest sexual enjoyment. The pleasure should always be mutual. If otherwise, something is at fault. For only one to participate is unnatural and little better than self abuse. The woman who is too nice to cultivate a passion for her husband ought never to have married. She incurs the risk of being deserted and cannot be pitied much if her husband finds more congenial society than hers. It must never be forgotten by a husband or a wife that ill-health, over-work and worry depress and even blots out the sexual instinct, while good health, happy surroundings and kind treatment develop it. No woman can have any great amount of feeling for a man who abuses her. If for no higher motive than selfish gratification the wise husband will treat his wife with the greatest tenderness. The various means taken to **prevent conception** are all more or less injurious to the health. The premature withdrawal of the male, called Onanism, is nearly as injurious as self abuse. Injections of cold water often cause long lasting womb troubles. The wearing of a cap of rubber or animal membrane over the penis is perhaps the least harmful of all these unnatural and more or less unhealthy measures. The false and pernicious idea that boys and young men, too young to marry, cannot live a continent life is doing untold mischief. It is sapping and dwarfing the average young man mentally and physically. Besides, he incurs the risk of acquiring syphilis or gonorrhœa, the evils of which have been fully described elsewhere. The young man who would be an intellectual and physical giant must remain absolutely continent the first twenty-five years of his life.

DISEASES OF WOMEN.

Besides being liable to suffer most of the diseases that may affect men, women are subject to a number of ailments that are peculiar to their sex. The most common of these, perhaps, are associated with derangements of **Menstruation.** The menses should return every twenty-eight days and the flow should continue three or four days, without pain. The menses should first appear about the fourteenth year and disappear about the forty-fourth year; lasting about thirty years. They may begin much earlier and do in warmer climates begin as early as the tenth year, or they may be delayed in a cold climate or on account of tardy development generally, until the eighteenth or twentieth year. They may continue to appear as late as the fifty-fifth year. The period during which the menses first appear is called puberty, and is accompanied by a change from girlish to womanly ways. The period during which the menses disappear is called the climacteric period or "Change of life." An absence of the menses after puberty and before the climacteric period, not due to pregnancy or nursing, is called **Amenorrhœa.** A scanty flow, a suppressed flow and a retention of the flow are included in the term amenorrhœa. Retention may be due to an imperforate hymen. The remedy is an operation. **Pulsatilla** and **Sulphur** are often indicated in amenorrhœa. When the flow is profuse the term **Menorrhagia** is used to designate it. A hemorrhage from the womb between menstrual periods is called **Metrorrhagia. Vicarious** menstruation is a periodic flow from some other part of the body in place of the menses. It is usually from the mucous membrane. Nose bleed is not an infrequent substitute. **Bryonia** is the usually indicated remedy for vicarious menstruation. **Hamamelis** and **Pulsatilla** may be indicated, also **Ferrum. Dysmenorrhœa** is painful menstruation. Naturally, there is no pain with the menses. The pain may be due to neuralgia, to congestion, to obstruction or to the shedding of the mucous membrane of the womb every month. According to the cause different kinds of dysmenorrhœa are named. Neuralgiac dysmenorrhœa is met in those subject to neuralgia or rheumatism in general; who are in a run-down condition. The pain is usually sharp, fixed and localized. It may begin before the flow and stop with its appearance or continue throughout. Ovarian dysmenorrhœa is due to a chronic inflammation of the ovary. The pain comes on between the menses, also a few days before and is relieved by the flow. The pain is dull, aching and accompanied with depression of the spirits and nervous troubles, also sympathetic disturbances of the breast. This form is often brought on by the barbarous habit very prevalent a few years ago among old school physicians of cauterizing the neck of the womb. Sterility usually followed. Congestive dysmenorrhœa is indicated by sudden, severe pains coming on during the flow, accompanied by a decrease of the flow and an increase of the temperature. The pain may be due to cold from getting damp during menstruation, inflammation about the womb, mental shock, excessive flesh in girls or displacement in married women. Obstructive dysmenorrhœa is known by the spasmodic pains coming on in paroxysms like labor pains. It is due to a naturally small canal or a contraction of it. It may be due to caustics or to a sharp bend in the canal. The pain in membraneous dysmenorrhœa commences with the flow and increases gradually, becoming labor-like until a membrane is expelled. The **treatment** of dysmenorrhœa depends upon the cause. In the neuralgiac form those remedies must be given which will correct the debilitated condition, while in case of the obstructive, the obstruction must be removed. The most general remedy in dysmenorrhœa is **Viburnum opulus**, given in ten drop doses of the tincture, every fifteen minutes. It acts more rapidly if given in hot water. It is particularly useful in the neuralgiac and obstructive forms. **Aconite** is often of great service in the congestive variety. **Belladonna** is indicated by severe, bearing down, throbbing pains, also throbbing headache. **Caulophyllin**, spasmodic pains in those subject to rheumatic troubles of the small joints. **Chamomilla**, patient very irritable, with drawing, griping, labor-like pains, followed by the expulsion of clots. **Cimicifuga**, rheumatic or neuralgiac pains. **Cocculus**, scanty, irregular, painful menstration, with cramps. **Gelsemium**, 1x, given every fifteen minutes in hot water, relieves that form accompanied by a disturbance of sight and the passing of a large quantity of pale urine, clear as pure water. **Pulsatilla** is particularly useful in suppression of menses after getting the feet wet. It should be remembered with **Aconite** in congestive dysmenorrhœa. **Silicea** may be valuable in chronic cases, where there is an unhealthy skin and an offensive sweat of the feet and an icy coldness of the body.

Displacement of the womb is perhaps the next most frequent complaint connected with the female sexual system. Displacement may be forward, backward, downward or sidewise. When the entire womb is displaced it is called a *version*, but if it is only bent upon itself it is a *flexion*. Thus, we have anteversion and retroversion, anteflexion and retroflexion. In case of anteversion the body of the womb lies too far forward and the neck too far backward. In retroversion just the opposite condition exists. In anteflexion the body of the womb is bent forward, while in retroflexion it is bent backward. A displacement of the womb downward is called prolapsus or "falling of the womb."

The symptoms of retroversion and retroflexion are very similar, except that the very frequent and sometimes painful micturition is much more common in the former than in the latter. In each there is a backache, a heavy feeling at the lower part of the abdomen, inability to walk any distance and going up or down stairs is particularly fatiguing. Inability to walk any distance is quite a reliable symptom of displacement. Spinal irritation and severe headache before menses also point to a displacement of the body of the womb backward.

The symptoms of anteversion and anteflexion are much the same. Backache and rectal irritation, however, are much more frequent in the former than in the latter. Both are accompanied with irritation of the bladder, difficulty in walking, dysmenorrhœa, sterility and leucorrhœa. There are three degrees of falling of the womb. In the first the symptoms are much like those of retroversion. In the second, there is much irritation of the bladder and rectum. In the third, a part of the womb appears externally. Inversion of the womb is the condition when it is turned inside out. It may happen during confinement or it may be brought about by a polypus. Displacement of the ovaries is a common trouble. It is indicated by pain radiating in different directions, by pain during intercourse and by pain during an evacuation of the bowels. Many displacements of the womb cause no inconvenience. Absolute rest in bed during the menstrual period is an important factor in the **treatment** of any displacement. Mechanical means to support the womb in its natural place are often necessary, though frequently abused. Proper rest, proper exercise and last, but not least, proper dress will do much to correct displacements. Massage and electricity are also of great value. Among the internal remedies that tend to restore the womb to its normal condition and position are: **Belladonna,** indicated when back aches as if broken and a bearing down as if everything would fall out. **Secale,** displacements following confinement. **Sepia,** in prolapsus. **Nux,** in many forms, and **Sulphur,** in all forms. **Calcarea Carb, Conium, Ferrum Iodide, Helonias** and **Platina** should also be studied. Each one of these is a favorite remedy of some physician. A tampon, consisting of a wad of cotton soaked with glycerine and inserted overnight into the vagina close up against the neck of the womb, will extract a vast amount of fluid from a congested and over-loaded womb, relieving it of some of its excessive weight so that its ligaments may support it in its proper place. A string attached to the tampon will facilitate the withdrawal of the cotton from the vagina.

Inflammation of the lining of the womb is called **Endometritis.** Like inflammation of the inner coating of other cavities of the body, it may be acute or chronic. It may affect a part or all of the inner surface of the womb. The acute form may arise from cold, excessive sexual indulgence, unclean instruments inserted into the womb, gonorrheal infection and from acute infectious diseases. The chief symptoms are a heavy, dragging feeling in the pelvis, back or thighs, accompanied with frequent and painful micturition. A leucorrhœal discharge soon follows and may be so irritating as to cause inflammation of the vagina, the canal that leads up to the womb. The mouth of the womb is swollen and stands open with a plug of tenacious mucus blocking it.

Chronic Endometritis may be a result of the acute or it may be caused by a tear in the neck of the womb. It may also result from the prevention of conception or the induction of abortion. The affection is not usually accompanied by any particular suffering more than the dragging and bearing down sensation. The patient usually comes to the physician for treatment of **Leucorrhœa**, a catarrh of the lining membrane of the genital tract, analogous to catarrh of the nasal or bronchial passages. There are three fundamental causes of leucorrhœa: Anæmia, congestion and specific infection. The anæmia may be due to an excessive drain from child bearing and nursing. The congestion may arise from a torpid liver or local irritation, as excessive sexual indulgence or masturbation. The specific infection is either gonorrhœa or syphilis. Leucorrhœa may be from the vulva, the vagina, or from the womb. The first is cheesy like, and seldom profuse. The second is milky and alkaline. The third is also, as a rule, alkaline, but not always. Leucorrhœa from the neck of the womb is thick and gelatinous, while that from the cavity, is thinner and more like mucus. Gonorrhœal or syphilitic leucorrhœa is usually acid; a nice point of distinction. The microscope will also reveal the germs of gonorrhœa. They may be present in the discharge a year after the disease was contracted and sufficiently vigorous to communicate it.

When there is a very offensive, watery discharge from the womb, which is sometimes bloody, an examination for cancer should be made. Whatever the form of leucorrhœa its **treatment** depends upon the cause. The anæmic patient must be built up by good food, by rest, by out door exercise, by a visit away from home and by salt sponge baths, with vigorous rubbing.

A leucorrhœal discharge contains a great amount of albumen and anæmia is a natural result of its continual escape. A nourishing diet of lean beef, mutton, eggs, cheese and milk is necessary to make up for the loss. Injections of very hot water night and morning are highly beneficial in acute endometritis, of which leucorrhœa is the symptom. It may be all the treatment, necessary. Chronic endometritis, however, is not so easily cured. Hot water injections may be beneficial or they may be injurious. In case of offensive leucorrhœa with itching, use Carbolic Acid in the injection. Five drops to the pint of water is sufficient; use Calendula for bloody leucorrhœa; Eucalyptus, for bad smelling leucorrhœa, such as accompanies cancer and Hydrastis, for a profuse yellow leucorrhœa. Open drawers and insufficient protection of the extremities during cold, damp weather, along with the constriction of the circulation by corsets are important factors in the production of leucorrhœa and the correction of these conditions are necessary before a cure can be effected. We have seen some of the worst cases of leucorrhœa, displacement and womb troubles disappear after dilating the rectum and removing all sources of irritation there. Many so-called womb troubles are secondary to rectal trouble. Dilating the womb is often beneficial. The following internal **remedies** are useful: **Tartar Emetic,** when the leucorrhœa is from the neck and body of the womb; **Belladonna,** when the leucorrhœa is due to acute endometritis; **Calcarea Carb,** milky leucorrhœa, with cold, damp feet and clammy hands; **Mercurius,** when there is a profuse, greenish yellow leucorrhœa, worse at night. The iodide is perhaps the best form of the mecurius in case the womb is enlarged. **Pulsatilla** is one of the best remedies for a thick, creamy leucorrhœa, with delayed or scanty menses. **Arsenicum, Kali Sulp., Lycopodium, Nitric Acid, Phosphorus, Sepia, Silicea** and **Sulphur** should be studied.

Erosion of the neck of the womb is simply an abrasion of the epithelium. It is often improperly called, by ignorant physicians, "ulcer of the womb." Ulceration of the neck of the womb rarely occurs, except with cancer. As a rule, erosion is caused by a **laceration** or tear of the neck of the womb. Sometimes a sewing up of the rent is necessary to cure erosion. In no other part of the body may a slight injury produce such serious symptoms as laceration. Continued irritation at the point of laceration is very prone to develop cancer. Various hysterical and neuralgiac symptoms may arise from a laceration; also anæmia, menstrual and even mental derangements. Operation is often the only remedy.

The following are synonyms of **Chronic Metritis:** *Areolar hyperplasia, Parenchymatous metritis, Sub-involution* and *Congestive hypertrophy of the Uterus.* They express a process by which the womb is unnaturally enlarged. Sub-involution is that condition when the womb is arrested in returning to its normal size after child birth. The symptoms vary, but usually include all those common to displacements and endometritis. An examination is generally necessary to determine and diagnose the condition. The patient should abstain from sexual indulgence and during menstruation should remain in bed. The chief remedies are **Secale** and

Sepia. The following may be indicated: **Belladonna, Mercurius, Sabina, Sulphur, Kali Iodide** and **Conium.**

Tumors of the womb may be benign or malignant, as in any other part of the body. A tumor which tends to return after removal and also tends to terminate fatally is called *malignant.* A *benign* tumor is one of an opposite nature. Fibroid and ovarian tumors, as a rule, belong to the benign class and cancers to the malignant. Tumors are much more common in married than unmarried women. This is particularly true of cancers. Profuse flooding is the most prominent and most dangerous symptom of a myoma or **fibroid** tumor. Very hot water injections have cured many cases of fibroid tumor. Electricity is also a successful agent in reducing them. **Calcarea Iodide** and **Secale** are the indicated homeopathic remedies. Fibroids, after the change of life, usually disappear of their own accord. Unless there is some special reason their removal by surgical means is not necessary.

As already stated, a thin, foul leucorrhœa, occasionally mixed with blood, points to cancer of the neck of the womb. In fact, 97 per cent. of the cases of cancer of the womb begin at the mouth of the womb. An examination should be made by a competent physician the moment there are any suspicions. Many a life may be saved by operating before the disease has progressed far. The only operation to be thought of is the complete removal of the womb. If done early the danger to life is slight and the prospect of complete recovery is good. A dark red or yellowish nodule on the neck of the womb, which bleeds easily, is likely to be cancer. **Arsenicum Iodide** is the most useful remedy in cancer.

Pelvic Cellulitis is an inflammation of the tissues about the womb. It is believed by some to be identical with **pelvic peri-**

tonitis, a localized peritonitis. Others regard them as two distinct affections, the former the milder. The following symptoms are common to both: Chill or chilliness, fever, pain, tenderness and exudation. The exudation is a plastic fluid, which solidifies and forms adhesions, sticking parts together that are not naturally united; perhaps changing the womb from the most movable organ in the body, naturally, to a fixed and stationary one. Recovery is the rule, although death may occur. One attack is likely to be followed by others.

Pelvic Abscess is generally a suppuration of an exudate thrown out during an attack of pelvic cellulitis. The abscess is generally accompanied by chill, fever, profuse perspiration, throbbing pain. It may break into the vagina, rectum, bladder or groin. It should be treated as an abscess in any other part. Open, wash out, disinfect and drain. The remedies likely to be indicated in pelvic cellulitis, pelvic peritonitis and pelvic abscess, are **Aconite, Apis, Arsenicum, Mercurius** and **Terebinthina. Hepar Sulp** may be given to hasten suppuration.

Pelvic Hematocele is a general term which may be applied to all effusions of blood into the pelvic cavity. The blood collects, as it were, in a sac and gives a tumor-like appearance. The blood collects as the result of a rupture of a blood vessel, due to lowered vitality and accident. Hematocele comes suddenly and is often attended with collapse and many symptoms common to severe hemorrhages elsewhere. The treatment is the same as in case of other hemorrhages.

Salpingitis is an inflammation of the Fallopian tubes, the connecting canals between the ovaries and the womb. The inflammation may be in the form of an acute or chronic catarrh and the result of extension of inflammation from neighboring parts especially endometritis following abortion and gonorrhœa, It will again be noticed that the evil effects of gonorrhœa are far reaching and long lasting. Gonorrhœal salpingitis is a common cause of sterility in women and may derange the tubes so as to render the woman an invalid for life. Salpingitis may have a tubercular origin. The symptoms of acute salpingitis cannot be distinguished from those of acute pelvic peritonitis.

Ovaralgia, or neuralgia of the ovary, may arise from the same causes as neuralgia in other parts. It may also be induced by profuse leucorrhœa, stone in the kidney, worms in the rectum, falling of the womb, tumors, erosion, laceration, retained fæces, irritation in distant parts of the body, excessive or incomplete intercourse or unsatisfied sexual desire. An attack comes on suddenly and is usually confined to one ovary. The pain is intense, cutting or cramp like, extending down the thigh or up into the abdomen. It has neither chill nor fever. It is better by hard pressure. The general **treatment** is much like that for leucorrhœa. The cause must be removed. During an attack hot applications in some form give the most relief. Injections of hot water may be given in the vagina and in the rectum. **Belladonna** or **Colocynth** may give relief. Valerianate of Zinc is highly recommended. The most effectual treatment must be done between attacks, giving whatever remedy is indicated. Electricity has done us splendid service in many cases.

Ovaritis is an inflammation of the ovary and occurs in an acute and a chronic form. The acute may be caused by child bed fever, suppression of menses, extension of inflammation from the womb or peritoneum, gonorrhœa, cold water or astringent injections, excessive sexual indulgence, abortion, acute eruptive diseases and the use in the womb of unclean instruments. The symptoms are very similar to localized peritonitis. The chronic may result from the acute or arise from poisonous drugs, displacements, cauterization of neck of womb, or from rheumatism which has been driven from another part by local applications. The chief symptom of ovaritis is a pain in the ovarian region or groin; dull, aching, burning pain, made worse by walking or riding over rough places. Ovaritis is always worse during menstruation. **Belladonna** and **Apis** are the chief remedies. **Bryonia, Colocynth, Lachesis, Mercurius, Platina** and **Thuya** may be of service.

It would require a volume, to describe minutely, all the various kinds of **ovarian tumors.** They may be benign or malignant. The ovarian cyst, which is simply a collection of fluid in a sac, is perhaps the most common tumor, arising in the ovary. It may reach an enormous size and collect several gallons of fluid. The surgical treatment of ovarian tumors is more successful than the medical. But little danger is now connected with the removal of an ovarian tumor of a benign character. A few cases of ovarian tumor have been reported cured by the use of **Apis** for several months.

The ailments of **pregnancy** are discussed in the section, Mother and Child.

SECTION IX.

Diseases of the Nervous System.

DISEASES OF THE NERVES.

An inflammation of the nerve fibres is called **Neuritis**. It may be local or general. To express the latter condition the term multiple or polyneuritis is employed. Localized neuritis may arise from cold, injury or inflammation in a neighboring part. While the multiple may be due to infectious diseases, organic poisons or debilitated conditions occuring from cancer, tuberculosis or anæmia. In case of localized neuritis a boring, stabbing pain is felt in the region supplied by the affected nerve. The skin may be reddened or swollen. The pain is variable. Numbness and a partial loss of the sense of touch may also occur. Multiple neuritis may begin with the symptoms of acute rheumatism or there may be no fever, but various paralyses occur, the most striking of which are the foot and wrist drop. That is, the wrist or foot suddenly loses its power and drops. In the acute form the disease may terminate fatally within ten days by the paralysis extending upward to some of the vital organs. We recall a case of a woman who had seemingly just recovered from an attack of peritonitis. She over-worked, apparently took cold and took some very strong medicine. There was at first numbness of the fingers and toes which steadily increased, extending upwards until it reached the heart and lungs on the tenth day and caused her death. She was perfectly conscious to the last minute and knew that death was coming. Her last words were: "Why did I ever allow them to persuade me to take allopathic poisons and desert my homeopathic physician?" The allopathic physician who gave her the strong drugs made another mistake in giving in the death certificate the cause of death, spinal sclerosis. The paralyses following diphtheria and excessive use of alcoholic liquors are due to multiple neuritis.

Neuromata is a nerve tumor. The pain in the stump of an amputated limb is due to tumors of this nature.

The **olfactory** nerve, the nerve of smell, may be affected so that the sense of smell is completely lost, or abnormally keen, or entirely perverted. Perversion is common in the epileptic and the insane.

Disturbances of the **optic** nerve are very often associated with disease in some other part of the body. A careful examination of the eye may throw a great deal of light upon the condition of the system generally. Bright's disease, albuminuria, syphilis, leukæmia, tobacco and certain mineral poisons are sometimes accompanied by optical disturbances. Meningitis and tumors of the brain are often shown by certain changes within the eye.

Sciatica is an inflammation of the sciatic nerve, the large nerve which supplies the hip and leg. It is a common complaint in those of a rheumatic or gouty tendency. The trouble may come on suddenly, but, as a rule, gradually. The pain, extending down one leg, is of a burning and gnawing character. It is a trouble that is easily recognized. It is often the result of some tumor in the pelvis. Rectal troubles frequently cause it. If due to any local irritation the first step in treating the disease is to remove the cause. **Bryonia, Rhus Tox, Ignatia** and **Colocynth** are sometimes of service in treating it.

DISEASES OF THE SPINAL CORD.

Affections of the spinal cord are so numerous and so complex that the scope of this volume will only permit a hasty enumeration of some of the more common and prominent affections. Injury, tuberculosis, syphilis and other infections are prominent factors in the production of a number of spinal troubles. A number of spinal affections are indicated by loss of sensation or over sensation in places and by inability to perform certain movements or by the presence of paralysis in certain parts.

Locomotor Ataxia is a common spinal trouble. Out of 300 cases of this disease there was a history of syphilis in 89 of them. Excessive fatigue, over-exertion, sexual excesses, exposure to cold and wet, are all supposed causes.

Sharp, stabbing pains in the legs, called lightning pains, are peculiarly characteristic of this disease. We were present at the bed side of a man with this disease when a paroxysm of pain came on so severe that the head of the thigh bone was broken off with a distinct snap by a strong contraction of the muscles of the leg. There is a gradual loss of locomotion from year to year until walking is impossible and general paralysis usually terminates the life of the victim. Want of reaction of the pupils to light and loss of knee jerk are early symptoms. These, along with the lightning pains, are sufficient to distinguish this incurable disease.

DISEASES OF THE BRAIN.

Headache, properly speaking, is not a disease; it is rather a symptom or sign of disease. Headache is a common accompaniment of a number of diseases. Disturbances and disorders of the brain, heart, stomach, kidneys, liver, bowels and sexual functions are often accompanied by headache.

In connection with the various fevers there is usually a headache. The exciting causes of headache are therefore numerous. There are, necessarily many varities of headache. Thus, we speak of gastric, billious, nervous, menstrual and many other forms of headache. Headaches occur in different parts of the head; in the front, in the back, on top, at one side. It may be a dull, steady ache, or it may be throbbing or piercing. One headache may be better when quiet, another when moving; one headache may be better out-doors while another is better in-doors. One may be better while lying, another while standing. One may be better after eating, while another may be worse.

Special mention should be made of a severe form of headache called **sick headache.** It comes in paroxysms and is usually confined to one side of the head. There is often associated with it disturbances of the vision. This form of headache is believed to be a hereditary, nervous weakness. It has been observed that it occurs in persons and families of a peculiar nervous type. When a person becomes mentally or physically exhausted he has an attack of sick headache. We are of the opinion, however, that sick headache is either caused or generally aggravated by some local irritation in some parts of the body, from the eye, nose, mouth, teeth or stomach, bowels or sexual organs. We have cured cases of long standing by means of surgery. Excitement, fatigue of mind or body, disturbance of the stomach, or the eating of some particular food often precipitates an attack of sick headache.

One of the striking features of sick headache is its coming in paroxysms. It may recur the same day every week, every fortnight or every month. Again, it may not recur with any regularity. The patient can often tell when the attack is coming on by the peculiar disturbances of the vision, blurring of the sight, flashes of light in zigzag lines. After the disturbance of vision the headache begins in a small spot with a sharp boring pain and gradually spreads over the head. Nausea and vomiting are common. The patient is very much prostrated; scarcely able to lift the head. The slightest noise or light aggravates the condition. An attack lasts from one to three days. It rarely occurs after middle age. Women are the greatest sufferers from this disease. This form of headache may be prevented, or the attacks rendered less frequent, by careful attention to the general health. Labor and worry must be lessened; more time must be given to rest and out-door exercise. All habits likely to produce it must be avoided, as well as anything that would weaken the general system. Many cases have been cured by abstaining from the use of tea and coffee. Other cases have been cured by the wearing of properly fitted glasses. One or more of the Homeopathic remedies mentioned below, selected according to the symptoms of the case, will either cut short or lessen the severity of the attack. Homeopathic remedies, carefully selected and given between attacks will tend to render less frequent their recurrence.

The treatment of headache in general is necessarily as varied as its causes. Almost any remedy in the Materia Medica may be found useful in some kind of headache. We will give indications for those only which are more commonly used and refer the reader to the Materia Medica given in Part II, to study those more rarely indicated.

Aconite.—Useful in headaches occurring in the first stage of fever, when the skin is hot and dry and there is great restlessness, feeling as if the brain would press through the forehead, dizziness on rising. Congestion of the head. Head burning hot. Sunstroke.

Arnica.—Headache or Meningitis, following an injury of the head.

Arsenicum.—Catarrhal headache; the head hot and the scald very sensitive; cannot bear to have the hair touched. Face pale and pinched. Thirsty, but dread to drink, because one feels worse after drinking.

Belladonna.—Violent, throbbing, stabbing headache. Pains come and go suddenly. Sleepy, but cannot sleep. Headache worse when leaning forward. Dizzy on stooping. Rush of blood to the head. Meningitis. Apoplexy. Dilated pupils. Boring of head in the pillow. Takes cold from every draught of air. Cannot bear noise or bright light. Worse when lying down.

Bryonia.—Head aches as if it would split, worse on stooping or on moving. Wants to keep perfectly still. Gets faint on rising.

China.—Throbbing headache, following loss of vital fluids. Brain seems to beat in waves against the skull, feeling as if the head would burst. Sleeplessness. Better with eyes open. Stitches from temple to temple; better by pressing. Headache better by standing or walking. Headache in the back part of the head ful-lowing after sexual excesses. Brain feels bruised. Ringing in ears, with weak, faint spells.

Glonoin.—Headache following exposure to the sun. Throbbing temples, feeling as if the skull was too small. Presses head with both hands. Feeling as if all the blood was going to the head. Palpitation of the heart. Blood vessels in the temples look and feel like cords.

Nux Vomica.—Headaches from dissipation. Loss of sleep. Irregular meals. Debauch. Intoxicated confusion in the head. Sight and hearing disturbed, feeling as if the head was larger than the body. Headache from sedentary habits. Stimulants; from strong odor, anger, worry and excessive study; irritable and nervous; feeling as if had not slept well.

Pulsatilla.—Headache after eating rich food. From overloaded stomach. From suppression of menses. From excessive study; from abuse of coffee and stimulants. Worse in the evening. Worse in warm room. Better in open air. Down-hearted. Disgust for fat. One sided headache.

Sanguinaria.—Headache begins in back of head; spreads upwards; settles over right eye. Better in dark room; must lie still. Periodical sick headache begins in the morning, increases during the day; lasts until evening; can't bear to have any one walk across the floor.

Cerebral Meningitis is an inflammation of the coverings of the brain. Syphilis and abscess of the ear are frequent causes of meningitis. Tubercular and infectious meningitis have already been described in another section. Fever, delirium, vomiting, convulsions, drawing back of the head, along with ear trouble, suggest meningitis or abscess. In meningitis the eyes are often crossed and the lids sometimes droop. The pupils are sometimes unequal. At first they are usually contracted, but later they may be very much dilated.

Meningitis is always accompanied by more or less fever. An ice bag to the head has a quieting effect. **Veratrum Viride, Belladonna, Gelsemium** and **Nux Vomica** are usually of service. Many other remedies may be indicated.

A congestion or an excess of blood in the brain is termed **Hyperæmia** of the brain, while the opposite condition is called **Anæmia**. The headache and delirium that accompany many diseases are probably due to congestion of the brain. **Anæmia** of the brain is indicated by fainting. In case of anæmia from profuse hemorrhages there is drowsiness, giddiness, inability to stand, flashes of light and noises in the ear. The natural treatment of anæmia of the brain is to place the head lower than the body.

Apoplexy is due to hemorrhage in the brain. As a rule, there are no warning symptoms. The patient is usually seized in the full enjoyment of health, while engaged in the performance of customary duties. Occasionally the attack may be preceded by numbness or tingling sensations. In some cases the loss of consciousness is sudden. In others it may come on gradually, several minutes elapsing before there is complete unconsciousness. The patient cannot be aroused. The face is livid or of an ashen-gray hue. The pupils are usually dilated. The breathing is slow, noisy and may be irregular. The pulse is full and slow. The urine and feces are passed involuntarily. The arm or leg on the affected side drops dead, while on the other side it falls more slowly. The cheek is more relaxed on the paralyzed side. The attack may occur during sleep. Small hemorrhages do not produce unconsciousness, but

Hemiplegia, a paralysis of one side of the body. It is complete when the arm, leg and one-half of the face are paralyzed. Partial, when only one of these are involved. If hemiplegia is slight the paralyzed parts may recover within a few days. If severe, it may require months. The leg usually recovers before the arm. If the right side is affected there may be paralysis of the tongue. Apoplexy is sometimes mistaken for epilepsy, alcoholism, uræmia, or opium poisoning. Hemorrhage from injury may produce the same symptoms as those produced by weakened arteries, as in case of apolexy, but the outcome is more favorable. The clot formed in case of hemorrhage by accident sometimes may be successfully removed by a surgical operation. Hemiplegia is common among children. In most cases the affection comes on with convulsions and loss of consciousness. As the child recovers consciousness it will be noticed that one side is paralyzed. The child may out-grow the paralysis or it may not. Mental imbecility and epilepsy may result. Children are sometimes paralyzed by an injury at birth.

Embolism is a clot of blood formed somewhere in the circulation and carried to the brain, lodging there and cutting off a large part of the circulation.

Thrombosis is the clotting of blood about an embolus. **Embolism** comes on suddenly, while thrombosis is more gradual. It is often difficult to tell whether the apoplexy is due to hemorrhage, embolism or thrombosis.

An ice bag should be put to the head and hot bottles to the feet. The head should be elevated. The bowels should be evacuated. Stimulants are not necessary. At first the limbs should be rubbed gently. After two weeks, electricity may be employed. After contractions have formed, electricity is useless. The prospects of complete recovery from complete hemiplegia are poor. The leg may recover, but the use of the arm is usually lost. If the hemiplegia remains three months and contractions form the case is hopeless.

Localization has been studied so that the exact location of troubles in the spine and brain can now be determined with considerable precision by the disturbances they cause in sensation and motion.

Aphasia is loss of speech, due to a disturbance in the speech centers of the brain.

Encephalitis is inflammation of the brain. It is usually the result of extension of inflammation from some neighboring part or from a distant part by the blood. Meningitis generally occurs with encephalitis. When due to an injury or an operation the symptoms may be acute, consisting of fever, headache, delirium, vomiting and chills, but when it is an extension from some other part, then it may develop more severely and extend over a period of weeks or months. Drowsiness and irregular fever are the chief symptoms. Its symptoms very much resemble those of tumor of the brain.

Cerebral Tumors are indicated by the following three persistent symptoms, occurring at the same time: Severe headache, vomiting and inflammation of the optic nerve. There may be also giddiness, convulsions and mental disturbances. Spasms of a single muscle of the face, arm or leg, with tingling, indicate the location of the tumor. Syphilitic tumors of the brain are the only ones that yield to treatment. Iodide of Potassium and Mercury are the favorite remedies of many, for syphilitic tumors. If the persistent headache yields by the use of these remedies it is good evidence of the nature of the tumor. A few tumors of the brain have been successfully removed.

Paralysis Agitans, or shaking palsy, begins slowly after an injury and is easily recognized by the trembling. It is incurable.

Acute Chorea, or St. Vitus Dance, is a common disease among children and is known by the irregular, involuntary contraction of the muscles. The patient unintentionally makes all sorts of grimaces and contortions. The disease is usually preceded by some debilitating disease or circumstance, as over-study or poor food. The disease usually yields to proper treatment. **Arsenicum** is often indicated.

Infantile Convulsions are fits or spasms, which involve the whole body. They occur more frequently in children. They may be caused by digestive disturbances, irritation during teething, rickets, fever, congestion of brain and infantile hemiplegia. A convulsion may come on without any warning, but usually it is preceded by restlessness, twitching, grating of the teeth. Usually begins in the right hand. The eyes are fixed and starring, or rolled up. The face becomes purple and distorted and the head drawn back. If due to indigestion or the beginning of an infectious disease, there is usually but one convulsion, but if due to intestinal trouble, there may be several. Convulsions arising from stomach trouble, infectious fevers and teething, are not so serious as when occurring from other causes. The first step in the **treatment** of convulsions, as in all other troubles, is to remove the cause. During the attack, chloroform may be used to relax the rigidity. A sheet wrung out of hot water and wrapped around the naked patient is a convenient and one of the most satisfactory ways of bringing the patient quickly out of the spasm. The bowels should be evacuated by an injection of water or glycerine. **Belladonna** is the most useful remedy in preventing and relieving a convulsion. **Nux**

Vom. and **Gelsemium** are also useful. **Veratrum Viride** and an ice cap may be needed if there is great heat of the head.

Epilepsy is a loss of consciousness with or without a convulsion. A transient loss of consciousness without a convulsion is called *petit mal*; with convulsion, *grand mal*. Three-fourths of all cases of epilepsy begin before the twentieth year. Epilepsy developing in an adult is usually due to some local irritation. The ascribed causes of epilepsy are heredity, alcoholism, syphilis, injury of the skull, sexual abuse, fright and local irritation. In case of **grand mal** there is usually a localized disturbance or sensation preceding the convulsion, which is called the *aura*.

The disturbance of sensation, or aura, may be in a finger or a toe, or in the stomach. An aura in a definite locality is of great diagnostic value in determining the exact location of the disturbance in the brain. The psychical aura consists of disturbances or perversions of sight, taste, smell and hearing, as odd sounds, flashes of light, unpleasant tastes and odors. The patient may scream and drop as if shot. The head is drawn back or to the right, the hands are clinched, the face livid, the jaws set and the mouth frothy. The tongue is usually bitten. The fits may occur at night and one be an epiletic for years without knowing it. The violent part of the attack usually lasts but a minute or two. The patient then drops into a state resembling deep sleep.

Petit Mal consists of a transient unconsciousness without a convulsion. The patient may be at the table eating when suddenly he stops talking in the middle of a sentence, the knife or fork drops, the eyes become fixed and the face slightly pale. In a moment or two consciousness is regained and the conversation is resumed as if nothing had happened. After the attack the patient may perform some irresponsible acts, as undressing or tearing up a book. Assaults of violence have been made, giving rise to legal questions.

Jacksonian Epilepsy is not accompanied with loss of consciousness. Prior to the attack the patient experiences a peculiar sensation in the face, the arm or leg. This is followed by a series of spasms of the muscles of the affected part, which the patient watches with interest. Many cases of epilepsy are and can be cured. The treatment must depend somewhat upon the cause. It is said, Julius Cæsar and Napoleon were epileptics. Children, with epilepsy, should be taught self control. Indulgence in whims weakens the moral force. We have seen hundreds of epileptic-like convulsions in male children cured by circumcision.

Five years ago an epileptic woman came under our care. After trying everything else in vain we operated upon the clitoris and rectum. She has not had a convulsion since. A systematic washing out of the intestines with three or four quarts of water has been followed by relief. A number of cures have been reported by each one of the following remedies: **Cannabis Indica, Belladonna, Glonoin, Calcarea Ars, Cuprum, Cocculus, Nux Vomica, Argenticum Nit., Œnanthe Croc., Indigo, Plumbum** and **Silicea.**

Neuralgia is a painful affection of the nerves, generally caused by debility. It may occur in the face, head, neck and arm, between the ribs, in the back, at the tip of the spine, in the feet, in the heels, in the stomach and other internal organs. Neuralgia may recur with a marked regularity. The treatment should be directed toward removing all irritation and building up the general health. For instance, if a decayed tooth is the cause it must be removed.

Belladonna, Gelsemium,. Arsenicum. China, Nux Vomica and many other remedies may be indicated.

Professional Spasms is a term used to express those affections following continuous and excessive use of a set of muscles, such as writers cramp, palsy of piano and violin players, telegraph operators, milk maids, weavers and cigarette rollers. Persons who write from the middle of the arm or elbow are rarely affected. The outcome is good if the part is rested for a sufficient length of time. The galvanic current is of service in treating such troubles.

Tetany is a paroxysmal or continued spasm of the extremities, occuring in those debilitated and otherwise deranged. The fingers, wrists, arms, toes and feet are all drawn inward. This condition may last for a few hours or many days.

Hysteria has been defined as that condition in which ideas control the body and produce changes resembling various diseases. It is commonly met in women, but may occur in men and boys. Heredity and education are important factors in producing it. Excessive study and the indulgence of every whim tend to develop it. Fright, love affairs, grief and domestic cares are among the exciting causes. Self abuse is also a cause of this affection in boys and girls. An attack may set in with alternate laughing and crying, or there may be a sensation of a ball rising in the throat. The patient may drop down as in an epileptic fit, but it will be noticed that they never fall into the fire or any where it will hurt them. They drop down easy, upon a soft spot. They may present many symptoms resembling a convulsion. But the tongue will not be bitten, as in case of epilepsy. The patient may present symptoms of paralysis and the case resemble one of true hemiplegia. In fact, there is no form of paralysis which the hysterical person may not imitate. There may be a "catching" breathing, such as is seen when one is dashed with cold water or as in brain trouble. There may be hysterical deafness and hysterical blindness. A hysterical cough may occur and has been mistaken for whooping cough. Even hemorrhage of the lungs may be simulated. The picture of all sorts of stomach troubles may be seen in the hysterical patient. It may seem impossible to swallow food. The patient may actually starve to death. There may be the most distressing flatulency. The patient may seem to have serious joint affection. But when they are put under an anæsthetic the joint is found movable and perfectly sound. As a rule, there is no fever, but some of the cases of high temperature that have been recently recorded, 112 to 120, are believed to be hysterical. Not the slightest dependence can be placed upon the statements of a hysterical person. They often deceive relatives, friends and physicians. One of the greatest surgeons in the world was led to believe that knee joint disease was present in a case. A young woman under our care, who had apparently been bed-ridden and helpless for years, was discovered to walk about nights as well as any one, when she supposed no one would know it.

In the treatment of hysteria harsh means are never justifiable, however provoking some cases may be. The physical condition should be carefully examined and congenial employment found. The bowels and lower orifices of the body should be examined. All sources of irritation should be removed. Electricity and massage are highly beneficial. The best results are obtained away from the home of the patient, isolated and under the care of an intelligent nurse. Hypnotism has been used beneficially in hysteria. **Ignatia** is often indicated in hysteria.

Neurasthenia is the term used to express a weak and exhausted condition of the nervous system. The symptoms are varied and general. The patient may be so physically exhausted as to be confined to bed. The least mental exertion causes a sense of great exhaustion. It may be impossible to add up a column of figures, and the dictation of a letter, a source of great worry. Trifles annoy such patients greatly. A trip abroad or a long rest is beneficial.

Orificial surgery, along with the indicated homeopathic remedy, will do wonders for many of these cases.

Traumatic Neurosis expresses the deranged conditions that follow a shock, which often resembles neurasthenia or hysteria. Hence, we have the terms, "railway brain" and "railway spine." A mental shock or a great mental strain may produce it. The symptoms may not develop for sometime after the injury or shock. The victim is nervous, irritable and changed mentally. He dwells continually upon his condition and complains of a great many things that would suggest conditions that do not exist.

Three years ago a sleeping-car conductor, whose car rolled down the banks of a Canadian railway, came under our care about three months after the accident. He would have convulsions to order and he could suffer the most excrutiating pain at various points in the spine when his attention was directed to them, but when his mind was diverted no tenderness could be found. He recovered after a year. **Hypericum** is often useful in spinal injuries.

SECTION X.

Unclassified Affections.

POISONINGS.

Alcoholism is an affection so common that it needs no description. Apoplexy, however, has been mistaken for it by ignorant police officers. The unconsciousness of drunkenness is rarely so profound but what the victim can be aroused somewhat, while the apoplectic patient cannot. Chronic alcoholism is best treated by confining the patient in a retreat, where the habits and diet can be regulated. Homeopathic remedies, given according to the symptoms, are of great value in treating chronic drunkenness. A person with delirium tremens should be tied in bed and closely watched, as they are very liable to escape. Several months ago a lady brought her husband to us at midnight because he saw snakes and lizards all about his feet. When he walked from his carriage to our office door he stepped so high in order to step over the snakes that persons on the street halted to see what was the matter. On sitting down in the office he saw a big lizard on the office chair. He complained of a wave-like sensation coming up his back and spreading over his head. We gave him **Gelsemium**. Within an hour he saw no more snakes and has seen none since. It is a disease and must be treated as such. The great attention that has been recently given to the subject of alcoholism will doubtless result in more successful treatment.

Thus far, treatment is a failure in many cases. We digress from our subject to say, that any young woman had better commit suicide than to marry a man addicted to drink. **Nux Vomica** and **Arsenicum** are often indicated in drinkers.

Morphia Habit is even worse than the liquor habit. A large percentage of cases are the direct result of allopathic treatment. The true homeopathic physician rarely finds it necessary to give morphine. Our old school friends are too ready with the hypodermic syringe as a panacea for every pain. The indicated homeopathic remedy will not only give relief as quick as morphine, but it will cure, while morphine deadens and suppresses. The successful treatment of the morphine habit requires the patient to be put in a position where he is under absolute control. The confirmed opium eater is sallow, emaciated, gray, prematurely aged, restless, irritable and troubled usually with itching. Except when under the influence of the drug, the pupils are dilated and sometimes unequal. Persons addicted to the morphine habit are notorious liars.

Lead Poisoning is a common complaint among lead workers, painters, plumbers and glaziers. The lead gains entrance to the system through the skin, the lungs or the digestive organs. Poisoning may occur from the use of cosmetics containing lead. Lead poisoning may show itself in an acute form in which there is vomiting, convulsions, epilepsy, delirium, neuritis and rapidly developing anæmia, or it may be chronic, manifested by anæmia; a blue line on the gums, caused by the lead being converted into black sulphide by the sulphuretted hydrogen from the tartar of the teeth; colic, its the most common symptom; lead palsies beginning slowly with wrist drop or spreading rapidly, paralyzing all the muscles in a few days. Inflammation of the optic nerve and trembling are common symptoms of lead poisoning. The arteries of lead workers become hardened, as they are in kidney and heart trouble.

Alumina is the chief remedy in lead colic. The following remedies may be of service: **Belladonna, Hepar Sulp., Nux Vom., Opium, Platina** and **Stramonium.**

Arsenical Poisoning may occur in an acute form or in a chronic form. When it occurs in the acute form it is usually the result of accident or suicidal intention. Paris Green or "Rough on Rats" is often the form in which it is taken. Shortly after it is taken there is intense pain in the stomach, vomiting and later colic and diarrhœa, with tenesmus. About three years ago we were called out of bed to see a young married woman who, as a result of a domestic quarrel, spread three teaspoonsful of "Rough on Rats" on a piece of cake and deliberately ate it. Half an hour later, when we arrived, she presented symptoms resembling those of cholera morbus. At a glance we saw in her symptoms the picture of **Arsenicum** and without delay gave her this remedy. An aggravation followed immediately, so severe that she confessed what she had done. The vomiting was encouraged, the bowels were washed out and large doses of dialyzed iron given. She suffered severely for forty-eight hours but finally recovered. Within six hours after taking the poisoning, cramping of the muscles begun at the toes and gradually extended upwards, taking in those of the abdomen, then those of the chest and finally those of the face. The contractions in the face distorted her features strangely. Her mouth was held firmly, several hours, in the position of one whistling and during this time she was unable to speak. Arsenic is used in the manufacture of a great many articles, as artificial flowers, carpets, wall paper, glazed, green and red paper. The most common symptom of chronic poisoning by arsenic is anæmia, with a pale, pinched deathly look.

Ptomaine Poisoning. In the decomposition of animal matter by bacterial germs, putrefactive alkaloids known as ptomaines and toxines are formed and sometimes these are highly poisonous. It is now believed that these products are the poisons in all infectious diseases. Cases of severe poisoning have followed the eating of sausage, pork pie, head cheese, beef veal and mutton. One day in July, 1891, four hours after eating veal and new corn, the writer was seized, while several miles from his office, with a colic which felt like ten thousand fine needles sticking in the intestines. It was accompanied by a profuse cold sweat all over the body and deathly palor. There was fainting and gasping for breath, also a feeling as if the heart was too large for the chest. As soon as his wife arrived she gave **Camphor;** ten drops of the tincture in a teaspoonful of water. Less than ten seconds the cold sweat changed to warm and rapid improvement followed. He was, however, confined to bed for a week, during which time he received **Arsenicum.** The sequel showed that the poisoning was so great as to cause intestinal hemorrhage and the loss of more than a quart of blood. It also explained the cause of the cold sweat and other symptoms of the collapse of hemorrhage. The case, without doubt, was one of ptomaine poisoning. Cases of ptomaine poisoning sometimes occur after eating cheese or ice cream, shell fish and fish.

Grain Poisoning sometimes occur from ergot fungus or by various poisonous seeds becoming mixed and ground with grain into meal or flour.

Accidental or Suicidal Poisoning requires prompt treatment. If the patient will not or cannot tell, a search of the house will usually give some clue to the nature of the poisoning. In case of acids, water containing salt or baking soda should be given. The white of eggs, as a rule, is beneficial in all poisons. If there is not already vomiting, it should be produced by mustard water. If the vomiting persists after the stomach is emptied, hot water and **Ipecac** should be given to reduce the irritability. If the poison be an alkali, as muriate of amonia, caustic, potash or carbolic acid (an alkali), give vinegar, lemon juice or sweet oil. Do not try to produce vomiting. If the poisoning is from an overdose of Aconite, evacuate the stomach and give strong coffee. If due to Arsenic, fly paper, Fowler's solution or Rough on Rats, give dyalized iron and a drink of mucilage or white of eggs. If Belladonna, give Opium and excite vomiting. If Corrosive Sublimate, give white of eggs and milk. If Digitalis, induce vomiting and move the bowels by injection, also give coffee and vinegar. If due to poisonous gases, place patient in open air, wash face and chest with cold water and give Opium. If due to Opium, Morphine or Laudanum, give strong coffee and Belladonna. Rub, whip and walk the patient about. We used these means successfully in case of a woman who drank an ounce of Laudanum and was unconscious six hours. If due to the poison ivy, give **Apis, Arsenicum** or **Rhus.** Bathe skin with Chlorate of Potash and apply Vaseline. If by

Strychnine or Nux Vomica, give tincture of Opium in twenty drop doses. For tobacco poisoning, give **Nux Vomica** and plenty of fresh air. In opium poisoning the pupils are contracted.

OTHER AFFECTIONS.

Sunstroke is a condition produced by exposure to excessive heat. Two forms occur: Heat exhaustion and heat stroke. Prolonged exposure, with physical exertion, may be followed by extreme exhaustion and collapse. The surface is cool, the pulse feeble and rapid and the temperature very much below normal. Persons whose work confines them to close rooms and who are not exposed to the direct rays of the sun may have this form. Heat stroke occurs in those who are exposed to the sun while working hard. It is commonly met in workmen in large cities who are exposed to the sun and who, at the same time, drink liquors. In this form, the temperature may rise to 107, even to 112. Death may occur within an hour, or the victim may drop dead, as if shot. It usually comes on with a pain in the head, dizziness, oppression, nausea and vomiting. Unconsciousness follows. Returning consciousness and falling of the temperature are favorable symptoms. The after effects of heat stroke may remain for years; the victim never being able afterward to endure with comfort a temperature above 80 in the shade.

The **treatment** for heat exhaustion should be of a stimulating nature. The patient may have to be given stimulants and be placed into a warm bath, while in heat stroke the patient is most successfully treated by being packed in ice. At least, the head should be surrounded with ice. The ice cap is the most satisfactory if procurable. **Belladonna, Aconite, Glonoin, Opium** and **Nux Vomica** are the usually indicated remedies.

Obesity is an excessive accumulation of fat and if not positively a diseased condition it is not evidence of the highest degree of health. It is often followed by some wasting disease, as diabetes. Over-eating, while not always the cause, is a common factor in the production of excessive fat; so is insufficient exercise and the drinking of malt liquors. The fat may be reduced by regulating the diet, taking more exercise and less sleep. If all the bread eaten be toasted and if all the liquid drank be hot water before meals, the reduction of fat will be satisfactory. Fat persons should eat meat but once a day and take starchy food in a limited quantity. They should abstain from the use of milk, coffee, beer cold water, sugar and potatoes. **Phytolacca** and **Arsenicum** tend to reduce flesh.

Ascaris Lumbricoides is a worm varying from four to twelve inches in length and is found chiefly in the intestines of children. The worms may migrate into the stomach and be vomited. They are, as a rule, passed with the stool. The child is restless, irritable, picks its nose and has a white ring about the mouth. Cold injections of salt water are recommended. **Cina** is the usually indicated homeopathic remedy.

Trichiniasis is produced in man or animal by eating meat containing a parasite called trichina spiralis. The embryo of the parasite lies in an egg which is embedded in the muscular part of the meat. When the meat enters the stomach, the gastric juices digest the shell of the egg and, as it were, hatch out the embryo parasites, which in the course of three days are full grown. They, in turn, within four or five days, lay eggs which go wandering about through the system and finally locate in the muscles, "the seat of election," and in about two weeks develop into the full-grown muscle trichina, causing an inflammation in the muscle. These, in the course of six weeks, become encapsulated; that is, three or four of them will become surrounded by a wall or layer and be completely housed in, as it were. Here they may remain for months and years until the muscle becomes meat and is taken into the stomach of man or some other animal, when the capsule is digested and a new generation hatched out.

Tænia Saginata is the common tape worm of this country. It may become fifteen or twenty feet in length. It is made up of segments. When fully developed the segments are flat, oblong and about half an inch in length and one-fourth of an inch in width. Persons usually learn that they have a tape worm by discovering these segments in the stool. Tape worm is due to eating infected raw beef. In Europe, a different form is common, due to eating raw pork. While writing this section we successfully removed a tape worm as follows: In the evening, after eating nothing but baked herring during the day, the patient took two ounces of an emulsion of male fern and pumpkin seeds. The next morning she took two ounces more, and an hour later a dose of castor oil. A two drachm dose of the etheral extract of male fern or felix mas taken after fasting and followed two hours later by a purgative of castor oil or citrate of magnesia will generally bring a part if not all the worm. The worm will continue to grow until its head is removed. The head is square and has four large sucking disks.

SECTION XI.

Affections of the Mind.

INSANITY.

In the discussion of insanity the terms illusion, hallucination, delusion and imperative conceptions are frequently employed and should be defined at the beginning. **Illusion** is a disturbance of vision. The objects seen by the patient are actually present, but are seen distorted and with attributes which they do not possess. In case of **Hallucination** the objects seen by the patient are not and have not been present. **Delusion** is a false idea or conclusion which no amount of facts or reasoning can change. It is the result of a weakening of the logical apparatus. Delusions are either expansive or depressive. A person possessed with an *expansive* delusion thinks himself a king or some important personage, or very wealthy, or it may assume an erotic or religious phase. While one afflicted with a *depressive* delusion imagines he has some incurable disease or is being persecuted, poisoned or pursued. *Genuine* delusions are those which have been created by the patient. *Spurious* are those acquired by the feeble minded through imitation. It is of great importance to determine whether a genuine delusion is systematized or unsystematized. In the former, the patient will present a number of arguments in support of his delusive idea, while in the latter, they can give no reason beyond simply affiming their delusion. For instance, if a person physically sound imagines that he has an incurable disease and enumerates a number of alleged symptoms to prove it, he is afflicted with a depressive, genuine, systematized, hypochondriacal delusion. If he is unable to give any reason for his belief then his delusion is unsystematized and he is in the first stage of paretic dementia or melancholia.

Imperative Conceptions are false ideas that occur to the insane, but they are able to reason themselves out of them and at times realize their absurdity, yet they influence them. They are seized with the morbid impulse to kill, to steal or to burn, just as a sane person is sometimes moved to jump out of a window or from a roof.

Insanity is not a disease, but a symptom which may arise from several different morbid conditions of the brain, the organ of the mind. All cases of insanity may be divided into two groups: **Pure** Insanities and **Complicating** Insanities. To the first group belong all those cases in which the insanity was the most prominent ailment of the patient and the *first* to develop. The second group includes those cases in which the insanity is the result of and *secondary* to some other disease, occurring *first* in some part of the body other than the brain. Of the *pure* insanities two great classes are recognized. One class, **Simple Insanity**, includes all those mental disorders which affect persons of a previously sound mind just as lung fever may a person who previously had sound lungs and had been perfectly well. The other class, **Constitutional** Insanity, comprises those cases which are the outgrowth of a previously weakened condition of the brain and nerves; due to heredity, infantile brain disease, injuries of the skull or the use of narcotics. Of the twenty-two kinds of pure insanities, fifteen belong to the first division, simple insanity, and seven to the second, constitutional insanity. Simple insanity is divided into two classes. To one, belong those cases in which no organic change of the brain can be discovered. To the other, those in which active organic changes may be discovered. To the first class, belong the following: Simple Mania, Simple Melancholia, Katatonia, Transitory Frenzy, Stuporous Insanity, Primary Confusional Insanity, Primary Deterioration, Secondary Confusional Insanity, Terminal Dementia, also Senile Dementia and the Insanity of Pubescence. To this class of simple insanity belong most of the curable cases. To the second class belong the following: Paretic Dementia, Syphilitic Dementia, Delirium Grave and Dementia from Coarse Brain Disease, such as tumors, hemorrhages or meningitis. Constitutional Insanity includes the following: Alcoholic Insanity, Hysterical Insanity, Epileptic Insanity, Periodical Insanity, Idiocy, Cretinism and Monomania. The Complicating Insanities, those in which the insanity is *secondary* to some other disease, may be classified as follows: Traumatic, Choreic, Post-febrile, Rheumatic, Gouty, Phthisical, Sympathetic and Pellagrous. Space will not allow us to define each one of the above forms of insanity. Only a few of the most common can be noticed.

Mania is an exalted state in which all restraints are removed and the mental faculties are exceedingly active. In short, at first the maniac resembles a person slightly intoxicated, and when the disease has progressed he is like one considerably intoxicated. He cannot bear contradiction. He laughs without cause and cries without reason, or raves with anger at the slightest interruption.

Melancholia is characterized by mental and physical depression. While every expression of the maniac shows exaltation, every look and act of the melancholiac reveals sadness and suffering. While the maniac indulges in ambitious schemes or contemplates with satisfaction his own greatness, the melancholiac broods over and is overwhelmed by his worthlessness and sinfulness; perhaps commits suicide.

Senile Dementia is a degree of mental enfeeblement in old age, greater than natural. Senile demerits very often claim that they have been robbed and will often place their money or property in the hands of any one but their friends. They lose their way on the streets. Do not recognize their homes. Roam about the house at night watching for thieves. Trembling is an invariable symptom of senile dementia. A few months ago the writer was called upon to give expert testimony as to the sanity of a man sixty-eight years old who had deliberately murdered his wife by stabbing her thirty-eight times while she was asleep. He had deliberately planned the murder. Days before, he had purchased the dagger for the express purpose of killing her. He bided his time and in midday, when all the children were away, he committed the deed. He then proceeded to the police station and gave himself up. Indignation ran high. Every one said he ought to hang. Even his lawyers felt so and had no hopes of saving him from the gallows. But when the trial came and all the testimony taken in regard to all his peculiarities, the judge and jury readily accepted our diagnosis of senile dementia and sent him to an asylum.

Paretic Dementia is dependent upon some organic change

in the brain and is marked first by absent mindedness, in which the patient can't tell what he was thinking about. Later the gait becomes tottering; the hand-writing, irregular; the spelling, incorrect; the morals, loose; the sense of honor, blunted, and indecent exposure of the person, common.

Chronic Hysterical Insanity makes the patient changeable, emotional, fretful, careless and superficial in their behavior and thoughts; they are vain, egotistical and desirous of notoriety or sympathy or both.

Periodical Insanity is a mental disorder which recurs after more or less regular intervals. Its recurrence may be associated with menstruation, hence the term, menstrual insanity, has been sometimes used. It may also arise from an injury to the skull or from alcoholic excesses. Dipsomania is a species of periodical insanity; the patient is seized with a desire for drink, which overrules every restraint and all sense of decency, for a debauch. Kleptomania is also a variety of periodical insanity, in which the morbid impulse is to steal. Some patients with periodical insanity have mania and melancholia in alternation. To this combination the term, circular insanity, is sometimes applied. Periodical insanities are more common in females than males.

Monomania, or paranoia, as more commonly called, is characterized by a fixed delusion, usually of persecution or of being wronged. The continual harping upon one subject is believed to be a prominent factor in producing monomania.

A physician will be more successful in examining a supposed insane person by presenting himself as a physician. Most insane patients are communicative. If not, their looks reveal their insanity. The chronic insane often have their pockets filled with bits of paper, tin foil and other things equally valueless.

A delusion is not sufficient proof of insanity. If it be accompanied with trembling of the outspread fingers and a difference in the size of the pupils, the presumption of insanity is strong; pointing also to the variety known as paretic dementia. Systematized, fixed delusions, are only found in monomania and hysterical insanity. Persons suffering from insanity following a fever usually recover in the course of a few weeks. During pregnancy and after confinement, mania sometimes occur, and acts of violence may be done. Recovery is the rule. Anger, fright and excessive joy have often led to insanity. Intellectual labor is rarely a cause of insanity. Proper mental labor is one of the best preventives of insanity. Self abuse and excessive sexual indulgence have been properly regarded from time immemorial as frequent causes of insanity.

The treatment of insanity by homeopathy is much more satisfactory than by the old way. The statistics from those insane asylums in New York, Massachusetts and Minnesota, in which the patients receive homeopathic treatment exclusively, show two and three times as many recoveries as do those from asylums in charge of the allopathic school. No doubt but what there are now thousands of persons confined as incurable who could be cured by homeopathic treatment. Orificial surgery has already to its credit the cure of a great many cases of insanity. Three, under our care within a year. Rest, massage, exercise, electricity, amusements and a nourishing diet are important in the successful treatment of the insane. A large number of homeopathic remedies may be useful, but the following are some of the most common with their most prominent indications:

Aurum, suicidal tendency; hypochrondriasis; religious melancholy. **Ignatia,** silent grief. **Kali Phos,** weeps a great deal from religious melancholy. **Pulsatilla,** weeps, prays and laments. **Lycopodium,** full of ungrounded fears. **Nux Vomica,** afraid of coming to want; quarrelsome. **Belladonna,** starts eas'ly; strikes, bites and attempts to run away; gay, merry craziness; suicidal mania; child bed mania. **Natrum Mur,** dwells on past unpleasant occurrences. **Cimicifuga,** sobs and cries; imagines the whole world against her. **Phosphorus,** extreme melancholy; loathes life. **Stramonium,** talks constantly; gay, dances, laughs and sings; is obscene. **Hyoscyamus,** wants to go naked, filthy in habits; complete loss of all modesty. **Anacardium,** incipient dementia; becomes profane; stupid and childish. **Aconite,** acute mania; fearful and apprehensive; result of fright.

"**Blues.**" Many sane persons experience a depressed, gloomy feeling which is often due to errors of diet or some other indiscretion. A light diet and a cold sponge bath before breakfast or a hot bath before retiring will do much to overcome it. Home-sick feeling and inclination to weep will often disappear after a few doses of **Pulsatilla** or **Phosphoric Acid.** Pleasant employment drives away "blues." A good diversion of the mind is to clean up and arrange one's room, trunks, drawers and books.

SECTION XII.

Diseases of the Skin.

SYMPTOMS.

The **objective** symptoms of cutaneous diseases are classified as follows: *Primary:* Macules, papules, tubercules, wheals, tumors, vesicles, blebs and pustules. *Secondary:* Scales, crusts, excoriations, fissures, ulcers, scars and stains. Macules are spots of discoloration on the skin without elevation or depression. Freckles and moth patches are examples of macules. Papules are pimples; a small, pointed, circumscribed, solid elevation, situated superficially on the skin. Tubercules are small, solid, deep-seated swellings about the size of a pea. Wheals are whitish or pinkish elevations of a transient nature. The swelling following a bee sting or nettle poisoning is an example of a wheal. Tumors are soft or firm elevations, usually large and prominent. Vesicles are small circumscribed elevations filled with a watery, cloudy fluid, the serum of the blood. Fever blisters are examples of vesicles. Blebs are the same as vesicles, only that they are much larger; may be from the size of a pea to that of an egg. Blebs are seen in case of ivy poisoning. Pustules are circumscribed elevations containing pus. Of the secondary objective symptoms, scales, crusts, also called scabs and scars, also called cicatrices, are so familiar as to need no description. Excoriations are the result of a superficial peeling off of the skin by an injury, as a scratch. Fissures are cracks, such as seen in chapped hands or lips. Ulcers are spots where not only the skin, but the sub-cutaneous tissue is lost from disease. Stains are discolorations left by a cutaneous disease.

An eruption is said to be confluent when the parts that compose it become so numerous and so close as to present one continuous eruptive surface. Discrete, when there remains patches of healthy skin between the parts of the eruption.

The **subjective** symptoms are those which cannot be seen, but are felt by the patient; itching, tingling, burning, pain, tenderness and heat; over sensitiveness and deficient sensation.

The **causes** of skin troubles may be divided into internal and external. Among the internal causes are heredity, constitutional tendencies, organic or functional diseases of the internal organs, age and sex, certain articles of food and drug poisoning. The external causes are climatic influences, irritants and parasites.

Diseases of the stomach, bowels, liver, kidneys and womb are common causes of a number of skin troubles.

There are eight general classes of skin troubles: (1). Disorders of the glands. (2). Inflammations. (3). Hemorrhages. (4.) Hypertrophies. (5). Atrophies. (6). New Growths. (7). Neuroses. (8). Parasitic Affections.

The following seventeen skin diseases are the most common and represent 81 per cent. of all skin troubles. They are named in the order of their frequency. The figures following each represents the percentage of its frequency of occurrence: Eczema, 30.4; syphilis cutanea, 11.2; acne, 7.3; pediculosis, 4; psoriasis, 3.3; ring worm, 3.2; dermatitis, 2.6; scabies, 26; urticaria, 2.5; pruritus, 2.1; seborrhœa, 2.1; herpes simplex, 1.7; favus, 1.7; impetigo, 1.4; herpes zoster, 1.2; verruca, 1.1; tinea versicolor, 1.

The **location** of a skin trouble often gives some idea of its nature, as many have favorite localities and are more likely to be found in those places than elsewhere.

"The scalp, is the most common seat of seborrhœa, the tineæ, eczema, sebaceous cysts, psoriasis and alopecia areata; the forehead, of acne; the nose, of lupus, rosacea and eczema; the upper lip, of herpes and eczema; the lower lip, of epithelioma; the chin, of sycosis and tinea tricophytina; the angle of the mouth, of epithelioma; the ears, of eczema; the front of chest, of keloid and tinea versicolor; under the clavicle, of sudamina; region of the nipple, of scabies and Paget's disease; the side of chest, of zoster; the elbows and knees, of psoriasis; the interdigits and front of wrists, of scabies; back of the hands, of lichen and eczema; the palms, of syphilide; the buttocks, inner ankle and toes in children, of scabies; the dorsum of penis, of scabies; the scrotum, of eczema, psoriasis and chimney-sweepers' cancer; the front of the leg, of dermatitis contusiformis; the leg, if running around or lengthwise, of zoster; the whole body, of pemphigus foliaceus and dermatitis exfoliativa; and the flexures of joints, of eczema and scabies."

Eczema, or tetter includes thirty per cent. of all cases of skin disease. It belongs to the second class, inflammations, and it is defined as an acute, sub-acute or chronic inflammatory disease, characterized in the beginning by the appearance of erythema (spots of redness), papules, vesicles or pustules, or a combination of these lesions with a variable amount of infiltration and thickening, terminating either in discharge with the formation of crusts, in absorption, or in desquamation (peeling off), and accompanied by more or less intense itching and a feeling of heat or burning.

There are, therefore, four primary types of eczema, named according to the character of the eruption at first: Erythematous, papular, vesicular and pustular. All cases begin as one of these types, but may lose their distinctive peculiarities and develop into the common clinical or secondary types: Eczema rubrum and eczema squamosum, or the rarer secondary forms eczema fissum, eczema sclerosum or eczema verrucosum.

In the beginning an eczema is very often of an erythematous type, indicated by smooth, red, inflamed blotches. It may immediately become papular indicated by small, solid, pointed elevations or pimples forming, or it may become vesicular, indicated by the formation of vesicles, that is, small, circumscribed elevations filled with a watery fluid. If the vesicles fill with pus then the eczema becomes the pustular type.

Two or more of the four primary types may be found combined. **Squamous Eczema** is secondary to the erythematous or papular form. It is characterized by scales and a red thickening of the skin with a tendency to crack, especially if located about the joints. It is common on the scalp and runs a chronic course.

Eczema Rubrum is known by its red, raw-looking, weeping, oozing or discharging surface, attended with more or less red, angry, thickening of the skin. The discharge from the raw surface, consisting of serum, occasionally of blood, sometimes dries into thick, yellow or reddish brown crusts, so that the whole diseased surface may, for a time, be completely hidden. This is a common form of eczema and is usually secondary to the vesicular, pustular or other primary types.

Eczema is often a very obstinate and persistent disease and generally worse in cold weather. It may be due to general or local causes. Among the general causes may be mentioned gouty and rheumatic tendency, derangements of digestion, general debility, exhaustion of the nervous system, dentition and a hereditary taint. Among the external causes are heat, cold, sharp, biting winds, excessive use of water, strong soaps, vaccination, dyes and dyestuffs, chemical irritants and the like. All the causes, however, may be stated in one, namely: Faulty nutrition of the skin. Eczema is not contagious. The successful treatment of eczema may require both local and constitutional means. Among the general measures are: Fresh air, exercise, regular habits, plain, nutritous diet and the avoidance of pork, salted meat, acid fruits, pastry, gravies, sauces, cheese, pickles, condiments, coffee, tea, also beer, wine and other stimulants.

In case the itching is intense it may be relieved by the application of cloths wrung out of hot water. Bran washes, boiled starch or linseed poultice will give relief. A lotion composed of one drachm of carbolic acid, one ounce of glycerine and one pint of water is useful in pruritus where the itching is intense.

In chronic eczema benefit will often follow the use of a jelly made as follows: Boil continuously one drachm of gelatine and two drachms of glycerine in three drachms of water until they form a transparent mass. Then, add one drachm of oxide of zinc. When desired for use liquefy by heating and then apply with a brush. For inveterate cases, an ointment is highly recommended made as follows: Mix one drachm of the oil of white birch with one ounce of vaseline. Frequent washing retards the recovery of eczema.

The next most frequent skin disease after eczema is **Syphilis Cutanea**. It may show itself as a macular, papular (rarely vesicular), pustular, bullous (blebs), tubercular or gummatous eruption. The eruption belonging to the secondary stage of syphilis is often preceded by fever, loss of appetite, muscular pains and headache. They are usually accompanied by enlargement of the glands, sore throat, patches in the mouth, rheumatic pains and falling out of the hair. The eruptions during the tertiary stage, occurring a year or more after the contraction of the disease, is usually of a tubercular, gummatous or ulcerative type. They cover a limited amount of the surface and have a marked tendency to form distinct circles or semi-circles. Pain in the bones and decay of bones may accompany this form.

Syphilitic eruption is usually of a dull, brownish-red or ham-red. It rarely if ever itches. A point of difference between it and eczema. The first eruption usually seen in syphilis is of a macular or erythematous type and shows itself from six to twelve weeks after the appearance of the chancre. Unless properly treated it remains out from one to two months. The eruption is generally abundant, but the face, back of the hands and feet may escape. Compound Syrup of Stillingia and Iodide of Potassium mixed in the proportion of one ounce of the former to one drachm of the latter is a favorite Eclectic prescription. It causes a rapid disappearance of the eruption. It should be taken three times a day in teaspoonful doses.

After syphilis cutanea in point of frequency comes **Acne**. It is a chronic inflammatory disease of the sebaceous glands, usually of the face. It may appear as papules, tubercules or pustules, or as a mixture of these. Acne usually occurs between the ages of fifteen and thirty. The eruption is irregularly scattered over the face and may occur over the neck and shoulders. The papules, tubercles or pustules, which ever form it may take, vary in size from a pin head to a pea.

The immediate cause of acne is over-secretion or retention of sebaceous matter in the glands of the skin. The indirect causes of acne are indigestion, constipation, menstrual irregularities, sexual abuse, general debility, lack of tone in the muscular fibres of the skin, scrofulosis, drugs, such as Iodides and Bromides, internally, and Tar, externally. Working in a dirty or dusty atmosphere tends to block the glands and produce acne. The disease is more common in those of light complexion. It is obstinate, but curable, after months of treatment. There are a number of varieties of acne. There is also a form called **Acne Rosacea** that is quite different from simple acne. It is a chronic inflammation of the skin, especially over the nose and cheeks. Dilatation of the blood vessels in these regions is very marked and serve to distinguish the disease. We cured a case of this kind of four years standing by thirty-five treatments of electricity. There has been no return of the disease after four years. We have recently dismissed another pronounced case of acne of a pustular character. The patient had treated in vain almost continuously for four years. After three months of treatment with electricity, using the galvanic current principally, the face became smooth. During the first month, we evacuated daily from six to twenty pustules on her face. Homeopathic remedies and orificial surgery were also employed in connection with the electricity. The greater part of the credit of cure is believed, however, to belong to the electricity. A wash with a saturated solution of boracic acid is quite satisfactory. Facial massage is also beneficial. Washing the face with soap and water and then sponging with very hot water gives good results.

The fourth most frequent skin affection is **Pediculosis**, that local or general cutaneous condition due to the presence of the animal parasite, the pediculus or louse.

Psoriasis is the next most frequent skin trouble. It is a chronic inflammatory disease, known by dry, reddish, variously sized, rounded, sharply defined, scaly patches. It is most common between the ages of fifteen and thirty. Its favorite location is on the outside of the elbows and in front of the knees. It may be confined to the scalp. The face, hands, soles of the feet and nails usually escape. There is usually some itching, but it is not troublesome, as in eczema. The size of the patches vary from that of a pin-head to a silver dollar, and they may number from twenty to a hundred. At the beginning, each patch is a red, scaly pimple, the size of a pin-point or a pin-head. It increases gradually and in the course of several days or weeks reaches the size of a dime or larger. Then, it remains stationary for some time or disappears. Its central portion vanishing first. The eruption is always dry; another point of difference between it and eczema. Psoriasis is a very chronic disease; patches may remain indefinitely. It is usually better in warm weather. The cause of the disease is unknown. In some way it is dependent upon the condition of the general health. It is a common disease and met in persons in all walks of life. It is not contagious. Psoriasis is distinguished from squamous eczema by its history; especially, the way it begins, the dryness of the eruption, and by its sharply defined, circumscribed, scattered, scaly patches. The scales of squamous syphilide are usually a dirty gray and scanty. The patches of syphilis are coppery in color and rarely have scales; besides, there are papules to be found. The face, palms and soles of the feet are often the seat of a syphilitic eruption, but rarely, if ever, of psoriasis.

A distinguishing peculiarity of the full grown patches of psoriasis is that they give the appearance as if drops of mortar had fallen upon the skin. When the central portion of a patch clears up it leaves a ring. Two rings sometimes touch, making the figure 8. When the patches have healed they leave no stain or scar. The scales are of a silvery white. Rubbing with cod liver oil is beneficial. One drachm of the oil of white birch mixed with one ounce of vaseline makes a good ointment. The following preparation is highly recommended: One drachm of Chrysarobin rubbed up with one drachm of Salicylic Acid in one ounce of gutta-percha. It should be applied thinly to the affected parts with a brush.

Tinea Trichophantina is the scientific name for ringworm, a contagious vegetable parasitic disease, due to the invasion into the skin of the vegetable parasite, trichophyton.

Ringworm presents a different appearance upon the scalp, upon the bearded region and upon the body. When it is on the scalp it will be noticed that the hairs within the affected region, break off and leave a "stubble" like appearance and the swollen hair follicle resemble "goose skin." When it is located in the beard, the term, "Barbers itch," is often applied. The treatment is to kill the parasite and render the soil in which it thrives sterile by the appropriate internal remedy. The most useful lotion is one grain of Mercuric Bichloride to one ounce of water. The hairs should be pulled out. A Sulphur ointment is useful.

Dermatitis is a term employed to designate those inflammations of the skin caused by irritants, such as excessive heat or cold, caustics and other chemicals; also, those produced by taking certain drugs internally. Dermatitis traumatica include all those inflammations of the skin due to injury, including those produced by parasites, by scratching and by chafing from bandages and tight-fitting garments. Dermatitis calorica includes burns and frost-bites. Mild burns may be treated by applying Bicarbonate of Soda in powder or saturated solution. In case of severe ones, use a five per cent. solution. Boracic Acid is claimed to be even better than Soda. Dermatitis venenata include all inflammations of the skin due to contact with poisonings. Ivy poisoning is a good example of this variety of dermatitis. Boracic Acid lotion is also beneficial in this form of dermatitis.

The next skin disease in the order of frequency is **Scabies**, commonly called itch. It is a contagious, animal parasitic disease, attended by itching. The favorite location of this parasite is in the tender and protected regions between the fingers, on the under side of the wrist, in the arm pits, about the nipples of females, about the privates and anus and the thigh. The face and scalp is not, as a rule, invaded. The eruption may be in the form of vesicles, papules and pustules. The disease is highly contagious and is most commonly contracted by sleeping with those affected or by occupying a bed in which they have slept. Burrows are twisted, straight or zig-zag, dotted, slightly elevated, dark gray or blackish thread like formations, varying from one-eighth to one-half inch in length, made by the female parasite burrowing a channel in the skin and depositing in its track fifteen or twenty eggs. The presence of the burrows is sufficient to distinguish the disease.

The treatment consists of a thorough scrubbing with soap

and hot water, followed by the application of a Sulphur ointment, made by mixing one part of Sulphur with eight parts of vaseline, plain cosmoline or lard.

Urticaria is next in the order of frequency. It includes hives and nettle rash. It consists of wheals, that is, evanescent whitish, pinkish or reddish elevations, variable in size and shape and attended by itching, stinging or pricking sensation. It makes its appearance suddenly and remains but a few hours. The disease disappears and reappears in a capricious manner. It is generally the result of dietetic errors. The stomach and bowels should be evacuated by an injection. A lotion of vinegar and warm water will relieve the itching.

Pruritis is a disease in which the sole symptom is itching. There are no objective symptoms whatever. The parts, however, may become irritated by the patient's continual scratching. It is more frequently met in advanced age. It may be general, but is very often located about the privates and anus. It is sometimes very distressing during the last months of pregnancy. The disease is caused by a depraved state of the nervous system. It is commonly met with digestive disturbances, liver troubles, diabetes mellitus and uric acid troubles. It is also met in the insane. Pruritis is likely to be mistaken for pediculosis.

Pruritis tries the skill of the physician as well as the patience of the patient. Lotions of Soda or of Boracic Acid, or Carbolic Acid, with water, glycerine and alcohol, give temporary relief Or, Carbolic Acid may be mixed with lard, lanolin or petrolatum, may be applied. If the skin is very dry, to an ounce of one of these, from five to thirty grains of Carbolic Acid, three to twenty grains of thymol or ten to thirty drops of chloroform may be added.

Seborrhœa is a disturbance of the sebaceous glands, known by an excessive or perhaps abnormal secretion of sebaceous matter, appearing on the skin as an oily coating, crusts or scales. It is usually seen on the scalp and face. The oily form of the disease is indicated by an unnatural oiliness across the nose and about the forehead. Sometimes, it occurs with Acne Rosacea. On the scalp the disease is manifested by dandruff.

Comedo has for its synonyms, black-heads and flesh worms. They are yellowish or blackish elevated points in the skin about the size of a pin-head, due to a disorder of the sebaceous glands. If the skin about the black-heads be squeezed a cheesy substance in the shape of a worm will be pressed out. Washing the face with green soap and then steaming it will remove many. The successful treatment requires attention to the general condition of the patient.

Herpes Simplex is an acute inflammatory disease of the skin, known by vesicles from the size of a pin-head to that of a pea, occurring generally on the face or privates. This form of herpes is often seen on the lips after a fever; hence the name, fever blister. When the disease occurs upon the privates the term, herpes progenitalis, is used to designate it. When occurring in this region it shows a disposition to recur. The disease remains for a week or two. Application of Spirits of Camphor will give relief, also a solution of Boric Acid.

Herpes Zoster, sometimes called shingles, is an acute inflammatory disease, consisting of a number of vesicles located upon an inflamed base along the line of some nerve trunk, such as between the ribs or along the back or over the eye.

The breaking out of the eruption is generally preceded by neuralgiac pains. The vesicles soon dry up, forming a yellowish or brownish crust. These drop off and sometimes leave a scar. The disease is limited to one side and is due to an inflammation at some point in the nerve. A mild galvanic current is beneficial. The patient must be treated constitutionally.

Some physicians oppose local applications and depend entirely upon internal remedies. They maintain that the skin trouble is only an expression of internal derangement. To a certain degree, they are correct. Evil may result from improper local applications. The disease may be suppressed and cause more serious troubles within. This is especially true of applications to the scalp. Whatever application is made it should be designed to accomplish two things and nothing more, namely, cleanliness and protection. Applications which do this and nothing more are proper and it is wrong to neglect to use them. Soap and water, pure oils, boracic acid, starch and Sulphur powder are always allowable.

Almost all skin diseases may be greatly benefitted by means of orificial surgery. A thorough stretching of the rectum, when it is unnaturally contracted, will improve the cutaneous circulation and consequently the nutrition of the skin. In general, all skin diseases are due to faulty nutrition. The curative resources of homeopathy in skin troubles are very great. The indicated homeopathic remedy will often make surprising cures, but may fail. In the early days of our practice, while attending a confinement, the husband offered us twenty-five dollars to cure him of salt rheum of the hands, a variety of eczema. We undertook the case. We have confined his wife six times since, but have not yet cured his hands.

The Internal Remedies for affections of the skin are numerous, but the following have a special action on the skin: **Arsenicum,** burning, itching, painful after scratching; pale, dry, bran-like scales; better by warm applications. **Belladonna,** hot, bright red and smoothe. **Hepar Sulp.**, unhealthy, suppurating skin; every slight injury maturates; skin very sensitive around ulcers. **Apis,** urticaria, sting of bees or insects; intolerable itching at night. **Tartar Emetic,** thick, pustular eruption as large as a pea. **Dulcamara,** nettle rash over the whole body. **Graphites,** itching eruption, from which oozes a corrosive, sticky fluid, looking like honey, in many parts of the body; excoriation of skin, especially in children. **Ledum,** eruptions which burn and sting, like bites or stings of insects. **Lycopodium,** itching, "liver spots," chronic urticaria. **Mercurius,** yellow skin; ulcer bleeding easily; base lardaceous; margins turn out, looking like raw meat; useful in syphilitic eruptions; round, coppery spots shining through the skin; useful in herpetic eruptions, also pustular eruptions. **Natrum Mur,** herpes, blisters on burning spots; white scales on the scalp; eczema in bend of joints; oozing acrid fluid; crusts with deep cracks; ulcers bleed and burn when dressed. **Nitric Acid,** warts, painful to touch, and bleed easily; fungus-like growths on the skin which bleed easily. **Phosphorus,** ulcers bleed on appearance of menses; blood boils; jaundice; dry, scaly skin; numerous fine, purple spots. **Phytolacca,** barber's itch; ring worm; syphilitic red spots; psoriasis. **Psorinum,** suppressed eruptions; eczema behind ears, on scalp, bend of elbows and arm pits; skin has a dirty look, as if the patient never washed. **Pulsatilla,** moles and freckles; measles; veins enlarged and inflamed. **Rhus Tox,** burning, itching eruptions; eczema, surface raw, excoriated; thick crusts, oozing and offensive; urticaria from getting wet. **Secale,** boils heal slowly; feeling as if mice were creeping under the skin; purpura hemorrhagica. **Sepia,** yellow saddle across the upper part of the cheeks and nose; moist places in the bend of the elbows and of the knees; brown or claret-colored tetter spots; herpetic eruption on lips and about the mouth; brown-red herpetic spots; moist eczema with itching and burning. **Silicea,** in females, violent itching of privates; eczema; ulcers, with thin, foul pus, sometimes bloody. **Stramonium,** suppression of an eruption or it fails to come out. **Sulphur,** the king of skin remedies, itching all over; burning all over; creeping sensations; voluptuous itching; nettle rash; itching hives; boils; skin rough, scaly, scabby; soreness in folds of skin; comedones. **Thuja,** wart-like excrescences on back of hand, on chin and elsewhere; warts, large, seedy, sometimes oozing moisture or bleeding.

SECTION XIII.

Diseases of the Eye and Ear.

EYE AFFECTIONS.

The **Lids** are subject to the same affections as other parts of the skin, such as eczema, cancer, erysipelas, abscess, acne or warts, and require the same treatment as when occurring in other parts. **Ectropion** is a turning of the lid outward so that the inner surface is exposed, giving it a red, raw, angry appearance. **Entropion** is an opposite condition; the lid turns in too much, so that the skin covering of the lid is in contact with the eyeball. **Ptosis** is a drooping of the upper lid.

Blepharitis Ciliaris is an inflammation of the edge of the lid. It is sometimes called blepharitis marginalis. It is caused by exposure to irritating influences, general debility, filth and by inflammation in neighboring parts. At first, the lid is congested. Soon it becomes swollen, shiny and smooth. Little pustules appear about the roots of the lashes and leave small ulcers or fissures. The discharge from these dry into small, yellow scabs, sticking the lashes together. The lashes often fall out. This disease is obstinate and has a tendency to recur. The local treatment consists in absolute cleanliness of the edge of the lid, the scabs must be soaked off with warm water several times daily and afterward pure cosmoline rubbed on the cleansed and dried margin. The internal remedies are **Aconite**, in acute cases; hot, dry and sensitive to the air. **Argentum Nitricum**, profuse discharge, sticking the lids together. **Arsenicum**, in chronic cases; burning; the margins thick, red and raw; discharge, acrid. **Aurum Met.** granulated lid; syphilitic or scrofulous troubles. **Calcarea Carb**, very useful in lid troubles of sickly children who sweat much about the head. **Cantharis**, very useful in chronic cases with hard, red, swollen lids. **Graphites** is perhaps the most useful remedy of all. Especially indicated when there is eczema about the face or head, as well as on the lid; moist eczema, with fissures and a tendency to bleed. Also very useful in a scurfy condition of the lids. **Mercurius Cor**, profuse, thin, water, burning discharge from eyes; lids, thick, swollen, red and sensitive; removal of scabs followed by bleeding. **Nux Vom**, lids troubles, with stomach troubles. **Pulsatilla**, very useful in many cases; cures styes. **Silicea**, no remedy more generally useful; removal of small scabs, followed by much bleeding. **Sulphur**, often useful.

The **Conjunctiva** forms the outer covering of the eye-ball and the inner covering of the eye-lid, so that when the eyes are closed it folds upon itself, making a shut sac not wholly unlike the shut sac of the pleura or of the pericardium, or of the peritoneum. Hyperæmia of the conjunctiva is a common trouble, due to overuse or abuse of the eyes by reading manuscript in strong artificial light or in a light too weak, by the bad practice of reading on the cars and by the worst habit of all, reading in bed by artificial light. There is no discharge, but the blood vessels, naturally invisible, become bright red and are seen to be superficial to and movable upon the eye-ball. There is smarting, itching and heaviness of the lids, worse towards evening.

To overcome hyperæmia, all injurious uses of the eyes must be given up and it may be necessary to wear carefully fitted glasses. Bathing the closed eyes with hot water or cold water to which has been added vinegar, or hamamelis, or salt, is often beneficial. Bathing with very hot water for five minutes three or four times a day will often be sufficient.

Conjunctivitis is an inflammation of the conjunctiva. There are several forms. The **Catarrhal** form is often preceded by hyperæmia. It is caused by exposure, eruptive diseases, injuries, bad surroundings, foreign bodies, contagion and over-use of the eyes. It is manifested by a sensation of sand in the eye, smarting, itching, watery discharge. Sticking together of the lids, mucus or pus like discharge. Lids grow red, swell and become stiff. The blood vessels in the conjunctiva become very prominent. The catarrhal form sometimes runs into the **Purulent**, which is indicated by a thick pus like discharge, which is highly contagious. This form needs the most skillful treatment. Absolute cleanliness must be observed. Towels, basins and other articles must be disinfected before being used by another. The eye must be cleansed every hour. This form is frequently met in new born infants and known as **Ophthalmia Neonatorum.** A large percentage of blindness is due to it. In some States there are stringent laws requiring midwives to report, within twenty-four hours, all cases of ophthalmia neonatorum. We have been successful by having the eyes wiped out every hour with a clean bit of old linen soaked in a solution of boric acid. A fresh, clean bit of linen should be used each time and great care taken not to infect the well eye in case but one is affected. We give **Pulsatilla** internally. Vilas says that one drop of a one grain solution of silver nitrate dropped between the lids night and morning, and a powder of **Argentum Nit**, 30x, every three hours internally, will cure all cases, if taken in time. The dangers of purulent conjunctivitis are that the cornea will become involved and ulcers form, resulting in sloughing and loss of sight. Gonorrhœal conjunctivitis is a variety of purulent conjunctivitis. It is the result of getting the gonorrhœal poison into the eye. It is very likely to occur in new born infants whose mothers are suffering from the gonorrhœa. Nurses taking care of cases of gonorrhœal conjunctivitis should exercise every precaution lest they carry the infection on their fingers to their own eyes.

The following case came under our observation lately: A man seventy years old, living alone and poorly cared for, bathed his forehead with coal oil to cure neuralgia. It set up a violent dermatitis on the right side of the forehead, which extended down into the right eye, causing purulent conjunctivitis and finally resulting in the loss of the eye. The left was saved only by a skilled specialist, Dr. Paul.

Conjunctivitis Granulosa is a granular inflammation of the conjunctiva, indicated by a peculiar roughness of that part lining the lids. It is often highly contagious. Some constitutional trouble usually accompanies it. It is met in those of indolent habits and intemperate in eating and drinking. If, in a case of conjunctivitis the up turned lid reveals the lines of meibomian glands down in the conjunctiva running to the border of the lid, like so many pillars in a row, the case is one of catarrhal conjunctivitis, but if they cannot be seen it is a case of purulent or granular conjunctivitis or something more severe.

Pterygium is a triangular shaped piece of membrane lying on the conjunctiva resembling somewhat a bat's wing. The base of the triangle is usually towards the nose, while the apex lies near the pupil. It is caused by exposure to winds and chronic inflammations.

The Internal Remedies for conjunctivitis are as follows: **Aconite**, valuable in the early stages of all forms. **Apis**, lids swollen and stinging, with a general appearance as if had been stung with a bee. **Argentum Nit**, its value, locally and internally, has already been mentioned in connection with the purulent form in infants. **Arsenicum**, useful in first stages of the catarrhal and granular forms; burning pains at night; attacks, periodical; shift from one eye to the other. **Belladonna**, useful in first stages, during hyperæmia and catarrhal form; useless in the purulent form; smarting, burning, dryness and heat. **Hepar Sulph**, in case of suppuration of the cornea. **Mercurius**, profuse burning, mucus and pus discharge; thin, acrid and excoriating discharges; conjunctivitis due to syphilis. **Nitric Acid**, gonorrhœal form. **Pulsatilla**, useful in all forms; especially, those following measles or colds; also, in infants. **Rhus Tox**, result of getting wet while over-heated. **Sulphur**, often indicated by the general symptoms.

The firm, dense, curved membrane which forms the transparent front of the eye-ball is named, **Cornea**, from its resemblance to horn. It is covered with the conjunctiva. In youth, the cornea is perfectly transparent, but in old age its margins become more or less opaque from fatty degeneration. The circle of opacity thus formed resembles in shape a rainbow and is named arcus senilis. The cornea contains no blood vessels except at its margin. Only in diseased conditions are they seen upon it.

Keratitis is inflammation of the cornea. It is due to inflammation in adjacent parts, bad nutrition, constitutional disease, injuries and exposure. The disease is indicated by pain, watery discharge, inability to endure the light, contraction of the pupil and impaired vision. There are two general classes of keratitis: Suppurative and non-suppurative. Keratitis may involve a whole or a part of the eye. Opacities frequently result. An opacity may be superficial or it may be deep. The former is curable. An opacity may be so situated as not to obstruct the vision, or it may shut out the sight entirely. The cornea may become so swollen as to burst, causing loss of the eye. This disease requires the careful attention of a skilled specialist. The object is to discuss it sufficiently to give an idea of its gravity. **Hepar Sulp** is likely to cure more cases than any other remedy, especially if the suppurative form. **Argentum Nit** is useful in the form following opthalmia neonatorum. **Rhus Tox,** superficial form, resulting from getting wet when over-heated. **Graphites,** when there is eczema in neighboring parts. **Mercurius,** useful in the superficial form, but not in the deep. **Pulsatilla,** in the pustular form. **Silicea,** small, round ulcers, with a tendency to perforate. **Spigelia,** sharp, shooting pains, with deep ulceration; eye-ball feels too large for the orbit. **Sulphur,** sharp, shooting pains, as if needle or splinter was being stuck into the eye.

The **Iris** is an iridescent, exquisitely colored membrane, the opening in which is called the pupil, hanging as a vertical screen in front of the lens of the eye. **Iritis** is an inflammation of the iris.

The chief causes are syphilis, exposure, rheumatism and extension of inflammation from other parts. The characteristic symptoms are: Changes in the color of the iris and alterations in the form and mobility of the pupil. The disease needs prompt treatment by a specialist. The treatment is necessarily internal. Vilas mentions thirty-four homeopathic remedies that may be useful, and there are as many more that may be occasionally useful. Besides all the remedies already mentioned in eye troubles, the following should be studied: **Kali Iodide**, syphilitic iritis. **Mercurius Dulcis**. iritis with corneal ulceration. **Bryonia**, iritis from rheumatism. **Lachesis**, pains in eyes and teeth; pains change from eyes to other parts.

The **Crystaline Lens** is a transparent bi-convex body about nine millimeters in diameter and three or four in thickness, suspended vertically in a transparent capsule, just behind the iris. The lens becomes harder and less elastic as age advances. By the same stages it changes from a colorless substance in youth to a straw color and finally, in old age, it is a brownish, amber color. It also enlarges with advancing age, but if it becomes cataractous it grows less. A **cataract** is an opacity of the lens or the capsule that encloses it, or both. The symptoms of cataract are a growing dimness of vision; distant objects look hazy and surrounded by a halo; later, vision for near objects is likewise impaired, and ability to see better in a dim light. On examining the eye sometimes a gray opacity can be seen filling the exact space occupied by the lens.

Cataract is not an unusual accompaniment of old age, but it may be present at birth, or it may be produced by an injury. It may occur in connection with diabetes or some other disease connected with the kidney. Cataracts are classed as hard or soft. The hard or senile is gray at the outer edge and yellowish gray at the center. They are usually uniform and striated; occuring in persons over fifty years of age. Soft cataracts occur generally in younger persons and are known by a lighter, bluish tint and are not likely to be striated, that is, streaked. The progress of senile cataract is variable; sometimes slow and sometimes rapid. May even cease to grow for a time. Senile cataract of one eye will sooner or later be followed by cataract of the other eye. Cataract may be produced by ergot, sugar, salt or alcohol. Cures or beneficial results have been reported from **Cannabis, Conium, Phosphorus** and other internal remedies, also by galvanism and massage. But senile cataract is curable only by operation.

When cataracts reach a certain stage of development they are said to be ripe for operation. Over ninety-five per cent. of the operations on cases of uncomplicated cataract are successful. The patient can then see by the use of cataract glasses.

The **Choroid** is a posterior covering to the eye and is somewhat analagous to the sclera or cornea in front. Diseases of the choroid are not easily diagnosed. Some of them may be detected by the ophthalmoscope in the hands of a specialist.

The **Retina** consists of a fine net-work of nerves, spread out upon the concave surface of the posterior wall of the eye-ball. It is simply an expansion of the optic nerve, and the mirror, as it were, which receives and transmits images to the brain. In the normal state of the eye the crystaline lens focuses exactly at the retina. In short-sightedness the focus is in front, while in farsightedness the focus is behind it. The office of spectacles is to supplement defects in the crystaline lens so that the focus of the rays of light will be exactly at the retina.

Retinitis is an inflammation of the retina. It is only detected by the ophthalmoscope. It may occur as the result of neglected hyperæmia of the retina, disease of the heart, or abdominal organs, pregnancy, Bright's disease, diabetes, syphilis or brain affections. An examination of the eyes by an ophthalmoscope often reveals confirmatory evidence of some of the preceding diseases. This is especially true in case of Bright's disease.

The **Vitreous Humor** is a jelly-like substance filling the space between the crystaline lens and the posterior wall of the eye. It is nearly colorless and contains about ninety-eight per cent. water. It is enclosed in a delicate membrane, called hyaloid. The **Aqueous Humor** fills the space in front of the lens and back of the cornea. It is nearly water. If evacuated, it will rapidly re-secrete

Glaucoma is one of the most dangerous affections of the eye. It is supposed to be due to the pressure of an over-secretion of the fluids or humors of the eye, due to irritation or inflammation of some part. It is characterized by severe neuralgiac pains over the eye, in forehead, temple, nose, with severe general symptoms, high fever, nausea and vomiting. In the beginning, the disease has been mistaken for typhoid, also for brain trouble. Before the onset of an acute attack there may be certain premonitory symptoms. A sense of fullness or swelling of the eye-ball, periods of dimness, increasing far-sightedness, pupil sometimes dilated. A halo or rainbow is seen on looking at a candle. The outer ring of which is red and the inner, bluish green. These premonitory symptoms may appear, disappear and reappear repeatedly, while the intervals between their recurrence grows shorter, until the acute attack sets in. Unless the disease receives prompt attention, total blindness results. About the only treatment is an operation called **Iridectomy,**

which consists of making an incision in the cornea and allowing the pent-up excessive fluid to escape. This usually secures relief and saves the vision. **Bell., Bry., Gel.** and **Spigelia** give relief.

Many eye troubles are dependent upon derangement of other parts of the body. Two cases of almost total blindness, which had baffled the best oculists, were cured by an operation upon the rectum. While on the other hand, disorders of the eyes may cause severe general troubles. Many a case of headache has been cured by wearing properly fitted spectacles, and a number of cases of epilepsy have been reported cured by the same means. Recently, a Chicago physician has made a hobby of curing almost all diseases by straightening the eyes and relieving the nervous system of all unnatural tension, just as other physicians are claiming to cure almost every disease by stretching the rectum and the other lower orifices. These hobby riders have some foundation for their enthusiasm, but they need the check of a judicial and broadly educated mind, to discriminate between the cases needing their pet treatment and those that do not.

In conclusion, let it be remembered that the homeopathic treatment of eye affections has been repeatedly demonstrated to be infinitely superior to all others.

AFFECTIONS OF THE EAR.

All kinds of foreign bodies may get into the ear. Great care should be exercised in removing them. Blind probing may cause serious damage or even death. **Inspissated Cerumen**, that is, dried or hardened ear-wax, may be found in the canal of the ear and should be removed as any other foreign body. It should be regarded as an abnormal condition. Its removal is often followed by great improvement in hearing. The presence of hardened ear-wax may be indicated by ringing, pain, sense of fullness or reeling and staggering. The throwing off of whitish scales from the canal of the ear indicates trouble of the throat and of surrounding parts. Discharges from the ear may come from the external part of the canal of the ear, the middle part or from the cavity of the skull. Boils in the external canal of the ear are very sensitive and painful. The best treatment is to open them and apply hot water. A troublesome eczema is often met about and within the ear. Applying hot water gives relief from the itching. The middle ear is subject to acute and chronic catarrh. **Acute Catarrh** of the ear is due to colds in the head, eruptive diseases, continued fevers, exposure to wet. It is indicated by a sense of fullness in the ear, hardness of hearing, noises in the ear, pain worse at night, dizziness and sometimes nausea and catarrh of the throat. Acute catarrh is an inflammation which secretes mucus, but stops short of producing pus. The milder form of the disease may be accompanied only by an uncomfortable stuffiness and a slight roaring, and but little deafness.

Chronic Catarrh of the ear is due to debility, syphilis, phthisis, chronic weakness repeated attacks of acute catarrh, diphtheria, scarlet fever and sometimes due to exhausting illness. It is indicated by a sense of fullness, deafness, dryness, cracking in ears as if air bubbles were bursting, noises of various kinds, scantiness of ear-wax. The earliest symptoms are the roaring and growing deafness. All the symptoms are aggravated when one is tired and exhausted. There are two varieties: One is distinguished by moisture and the other by dryness. The former yields to treatment much more readily than the latter, which is sometimes improperly called nervous deafness.

Chronic catarrh needs prompt and continued treatment by a skilled specialist. Delays are dangerous.

Acute Suppuration of the ear may result from prolonged acute catarrh, which always precedes it. In this disease, all the symptoms of acute catarrh are present, much intensified. The pain is very intense and is generally referred directly to the ear, though extending to the temple, eye and back part of the head. The pus will cause a bulging out of the drum head, something that any quantity of mucus will not do. On account of the Eustachian tube, the canal from the ear to the throat being closed by the catarrhal condition, the pus is shut in behind the drum head forming an abscess. The tendency of pus is always to burrow in the direction of the least resistance. Hence, perforation of the drum head is the common result, yet it may burrow through the thin bone that separates the ear from the brain and very serious consequences follow. The established rule for the treatment of abscesses in other parts holds good here. Make an incision in the drum head and remove the pus.

Hot water will relieve the pain. If the drum head has not been perforated the pain may be relieved by dropping in the ear a few drops of a two to five per cent. solution of atropia sulphate. **Hepar Sulp.**, useful in hastening and in arresting suppuration. **Arsenicum,** where there is great debility. **Aconite,** valuable in early stage. **Mercurius,** acts on Eustachian, and drum head. **Belladonna,** throbbing pain, wild expression, delirium. **Arsenicum,** also has great exhaustion, humming and loss of hearing.

Chronic Suppuration of the ear is commonly called

otorrhœa. Among the causes are: Previous inflammation and disease of the bones of the ear, diphtheria and scarlet fever. The disease is indicated by an offensive, purulent discharge from the ear. The canal of the ear is reddened by contact with the irritating pus. The first step in the treatment is absolute cleanliness of the canal of the ear. General treatment of the patient is usually needed. **Polypi** often results from otorrhœa. **Cerebral Abscess** may occur by the pus burrowing through the skull into the brain. Besides those mentioned for the acute form, the following should be studied: **Calcarea Carb, Aurum Met., Mercurius, Sulphur, Nitric Acid and Silicea.**

It is a common occurrence to meet persons suffering from some ear trouble dating from an attack of scarlet fever or measles. But, it is exceedingly rare to find such a case following homeopathic treatment of scarlet fever or measles. We have never seen but one. The amount of ear and eye troubles that have been and may be prevented by homeopathic treatment, is beyond comprehension.

SECTION XIV.

The Principles of Surgery.

MEDICINE AND SURGERY.

The relation of the field of medicine and the field of surgery may be compared to that of two overlapping circles. They have some portions in common and it is often difficult to tell where one leaves off and where the other begins, while other parts are so distinct that one could not possibly be mistaken for the other. If a healthy person falls and breaks his arm it is, unquestionably, a surgical case. A homeopathic surgeon was called several miles to amputate a leg that was covered with tumors. Instead of amputating he gave Natrum Mur. Within six weeks, all tumors disappeared and perfect use of the leg was regained. A man, some three weeks after an apparently light injury, had a severe chill followed by high fever. During the next four days, we used every remedy that could possibly be indicated. His temperature continued high and symptoms of dissolution threatened. An incision in the abdomen let out a pint of pus. Within twelve hours afterwards his temperature was normal and continued so. A speedy recovery followed. A celebrated London physician amputated one leg of an old lady for senile gangrene. The disease appeared in the other foot and he insisted on amputating that one also. But she refused and passed into the hands of a homeopathic physician, who cured her with **Secale**. No doubt but that the first leg might have been saved by the same means. Thousands of lives are lost every year for want of surgical interference in empyema following pleuritis. A safe medical adviser should be, therefore, a surgeon as well as a physician, and a physician as well as a surgeon.

INJURY AND REPAIR.

Whenever an **injury** occurs the tissue cells in the track and on the borders of the wound are destroyed, together with a quantity of blood cells, along with the serum. These are killed and are very similar, if not identical, with fresh meat. In the preservation of fresh meat, an idea of the fundamental principle of treating wounds may be gained. Fresh meat may be preserved from **decomposition** by one of three ways: Removing all *moisture*, as in case of dried beef. Extracting all *heat*, as in case of frozen meat, or in protecting it from *germs*, as in case of canned or salted meat. It is at once seen that three conditions are absolutely necessary before decomposition can take place. *Moisture, heat* and *germs*. If any one of these conditions are absent, decomposition will not occur. In the treatment of wounds, the preservation of the dead parts from decomposition is the first essential. We cannot remove all moisture from a wound, nor can we extract all heat. The only condition we can utilize is to protect it from germs. This implies absolute cleanliness and protection from the first until the wound is healed. It is only within the past five years that surgical cleanliness has been understood. Upon it, depends the success or failure of every important surgical operation.

A wound which is perfectly clean is called an aseptic wound. One that is infected with germs, is called septic. To disinfect a wound is to wash it with a disinfecting or germicidal fluid. The tendency of all wounds in healthy persons is to heal immediately. They will heal promptly without inflammation if they are not irritated. **Irritation** may be mechanical, chemical or parasitic. We are surrounded with germs that can only live in dead matter. They cannot live in live matter. When they gain entrance to the dead discharge from an open wound they thrive and produce a chemical poison, which becomes an irritant, producing a condition known as inflammation or wound fever. Wound fever or **inflammation is** the result of continued irritation, whether it be mechanical, chemical or parasitical. Inflammation is distinguished by redness, swelling, heat and pain. In addition to these local signs, inflammation is always accompanied by an increase of temperature and a quickened pulse. If very great, the respirations will be quickened, the appetite lost and all the secretions diminished. In acute inflammation, the temperature may reach 105, but in chronic, it is slight. The proper treatment of **wounds** at once becomes apparent, namely: Cleanse of all foreign matter of whatever kind and then put on an air tight or antiseptic dressing, so as to keep out all germs and then immobilize so there can be no mechanical irritation. An antiseptic dressing is some substance that is antagonistic to the existence or reproduction of germs. It is of a germicidal or disinfecting nature. The most powerful disinfectant is corrosive sublimate or **Bi-Chloride** of Mercury. It is also a dangerous poison. A solution of 1 to 1,000 may be used to disinfect the unbroken skin, but in washing a wound it should not be used stronger than 1 to 5,000. Salivation, dysenteric diarrhœa, vomiting, collapse and death have followed its use in too strong a solution. It is ruinous to steel instruments. It is generally used to wash out septic wounds. Bits of gauze, which have been boiled in a solution of this disinfectant, are now commonly used in operations in place of sponges, to soak up the blood from the wound. Wounds are often dressed with gauze prepared in the same way. Gauze, however, into which Iodoform has been incorporated, is probably used more frequently for dressing wounds. **Iodoform** is a yellow, horribly smelling powder, that is used very generally in the dressing of wounds. The common practice is to dust the wound with the Iodoform powder and then over it bind Iodoform gauze. The horrible odor is very objectionable, yet, we must confess, that we have not yet seen any other dressing quite so satisfactory. The Iodoform powder tends to check the hemorrhage or oozing from the wound and keeps it dry; a very important point, as we have just observed that moisture is essential to decomposition; germs cannot thrive without moisture. Iodoform is not such a powerful germicide as the bi-chloride of mercury, yet cases of poisoning have followed its use. **Carbolic Acid** is used extensively in surgical practice, but it is far from being all that could be desired. According to Koch, instruments to be absolutely disinfected, should be soaked in a five per cent. solution two days. One part in forty of water, is the ordinary strength used in cleansing wounds; one in twenty, for instruments and sponges.

Poisoning may follow its use, indicated by an olive green urine, headache, nausea, giddiness and great depression and even collapse. **Eucalyptus** is a good substitute for carbolic acid. **Boric Acid** is non-poisonous and may be used in a saturated solution or dusted on the wound in powder form. It is not so effective as other disinfectants.

Peroxide of Hydrogen is very useful to destroy pus. It has come into general use within three years. It is a non-poisonous fluid, resembling water, and may be injected into any pus cavity. It is becoming deservedly popular as a pus destroyer.

Suppuration, that is, the formation of pus in a wound, is generally believed to be due to the presence in the wound of pus microbes and that suppuration cannot occur without them. The pus microbe called, *Staphylococcus Pyogenes Aureus*, is the one most commonly met in acute abscesses, while the *Streptococcus Pyogenes* is the one generally met in such grave affections as pyæmia and progressive gangrene.

Pus consists chiefly of dead, white, blood corpuscles, debris of tissue and germs floating in a highly albuminous fluid.

White Blood Corpuscles are the natural protectors of the system against the germs of disease. When one of them and a germ come in contact the result is the death of one or the other. If the system is in a good condition the white blood corpuscle is generally triumphant.

An **Abscess** is a circumscribed collection of pus enclosed in a cavity of its own formation. Abscesses are either acute or chronic, according to the intensity of their symptoms and the rapidity of their development. The local symptoms of abscess are at first the same as inflammation. An ordinary boil is a good example of a superficial abscess. Pus is forced to the surface in the line of the least resistance. **Hepar Sulph.** either arrests or hastens the formation of an abscess. As soon as an abscess has formed, the rule is to open it. In case of **felon**, much pain and suffering may be prevented by opening at once. An abscess should never be squeezed. Abscesses should be washed out with some disinfecting solution. Corrosive sublimate is commonly used. But the great English surgeon, Sir Joseph Lister, has returned to the use of Carbolic Acid; disagreeing with Koch and claiming that it is the best and most satisfactory disinfectant of all; a half hour being sufficient time to disinfect instruments in a solution of 1 to 20. Deep abscesses should have a rubber tube or a strip of Iodoform gauze inserted to keep them open so that they may drain thoroughly.

Deep abscesses are not always easily recognized They may be indicated by a severe chill, high fever, throbbing pain and an inflammatory œdema, that is, a tender, swollen, doughy feeling, in the middle of which there is a soft spot.

Chronic abscesses are commonly called **Cold** abscesses. They are usually due to tubercular infection, but occasionally may be of syphilitic origin. The former is surrounded by a wall called pyogenic membrane. The latter is not. Cold abscess may exist for months. A common location is near the spinal column, due to tubercular disease of the spine. A slight elevation of temperature usually accompanies cold abscesses. In evacuating them, every antiseptic precaution should be employed lest true suppuration follow, by the wound becoming infected with pus germs as well as tubercular germs.

The greater success that now attends surgical operations is due almost entirely to **Antiseptic Precautions.** Before every operation, the skin over and about the region where the incision is to be made, should be thoroughly cleansed, as follows: Shave off all hair. Scrub with green soap and water. Wash with Corrosive Sublimate, 1 to 1,000. Then bind on and leave over night gauze saturated with Carbolic Acid and Glycerine and covered with oiled silk. Just before operating, remove the gauze and wash the part with absolute alcohol or ether. Towels saturated with a solution of Corrosive Sublimate or Carbolic Acid should be spread about the place to be operated. The **instruments** should be placed in a basin of carbolized water, 1 to 20, half an hour before the operation and kept there throughout the operation except when in actual use. After the operation, instruments should be plunged into boiling water and afterwards carefully wiped and dried. The **hands** of the operator and of the assistants should be thoroughly disinfected by scrubbing with soap, water and nail brush. All particles of dirt must be removed from under the nails. The hands should then be washed in a solution of Corrosive Sublimate, 1 to 1,000, or Carbolic Acid, 1 to 20, and afterwards washed in pure water or absolute alcohol. Nothing should come near the region to be operated upon without being disinfected. Bits of Corrosive Sublimate gauze are now generally used as sponges. If sponges are used, they should be soaked for hours in a solution of Carbolic Acid, 1 to 20. The water used to wash out the wound made during the operation should be thrice boiled and kept in an air-tight receptacle or jar. If the wound is septic from the presence of pus then it should be washed out with a solution of Corrosive Sublimate, 1 to 5,000. We have already described how a wound should be **dressed**. If large or septic, make drainage by inserting a rubber tube or a strip of gauze or a piece of cat-gut thread, leaving one end hang out of the wound. Then bring the edges of the wound together and hold there by stitches of silk or cat-gut or silver wire. These should, also, be kept in a solution of Carbolic Acid until used. Over the wound Iodoform should be dusted and then over it Iodoform gauze should be bound, covered with cotton and a bandage. The dressing may be left on from one day to a week, according to the symptoms. Increasing pain, soreness and fever, or hemorrhage or oozing, would call for a redressing. An idea of the marvelous progress of surgery may be gained from the simple fact that when President Garfield was shot, only twelve years ago, no antiseptic precautions whatever were taken. Antiseptic treatment had scarcely been heard of and the cause of inflammation and suppuration were unknown. That they were, in any way, due to a germ, had hardly been thought of. If the commonest citizen should receive to-day such treatment as Garfield received, it would be considered the worst kind of malpractice.

Anæsthetics are agents employed to render the patient unconscious or insensible to pain during an operation. The chief general anæsthetics are Chloroform and Ether. The use of both were discovered about the year 1844. Cocaine is the common local anæsthetic. It came into use about ten years ago. "Which is the safer anæsthetic?" is a question that comes up for discussion every year in medical meetings, just as the tariff question comes up at every Presidential campaign. Ether is generally supposed to be the less dangerous. But the recent death of a distinguished New York editor by this anæsthetic while undergoing an operation at the hands of two very eminent surgeons of that city, has again confirmed the fact that death may occur from either. To whom and how it is given are more practical questions.

Ether is a powerful irritant of the mucous membrane. It must not be given in case of lung or kidney trouble. On account of the profuse flow of saliva it produces, it cannot be used for operations about the mouth. Ether must not be used at night. It is liable to ignite with the lamp or gas light. Horrible cases of burning have occurred from this cause. Ether is said to stimulate the heart while Chloroform depresses it. Ether kills by suffocation; Chloroform by paralyzing the heart. The evil effects of Ether last for hours, even days. It may cause severe vomiting and is liable to rupture the stitches in case of large wounds of the abdomen. The vomiting may be controlled by giving coffee or a quick acting cathartic, such as citrate of magnesia. Infants and old persons bear Chloroform better that Ether. Death from Chloroform occurs on the table during the operation. Death from Ether may not occur for several hours afterward; even the next day, and be attributed to some other cause. There is no telling how many deaths do occur from Ether. But a death from Chloroform is always known. It is estimated that Chloroform causes one death in 10,000 and Ether one in 25,000. A mixture of one part of Chloroform and two of Ether has given us good satisfaction. The A C E mixture, consisting of one part Alcohol, two parts of Chloroform and three parts of Ether is highly praised. Packard, of Boston, is advocating the use of etherized air, consisting of a mixture of Ether and air, in the proportion of one drop of the former to one cubic inch of the latter. Besides economy and simplicity, it has much to recommend it.

Rules. Patient should not eat any solid food for four hours before taking an anæsthetic, nor any liquid food for two hours. The heart should always be examined. The urine should be examined before giving Ether. Vaseline rubbed over the face will prevent the fumes from burning the skin. The eyes should be closed for the same reason. False teeth, tobacco and every other loose article in the mouth must be removed, lest they fall into the wind pipe and produce suffocation. All constricting bands about the neck and waist must be loosened. The patient must be placed in a reclining position. The anæsthetic must not be crowded at first. It is well, in case of timid patients, to allow them to hold the anæsthetic until they become familiar with it. Both breathing and pulse should be watched. Shallow or irregular breathing calls for a temporary withdrawal of the anæsthetic.

In giving Chloroform, a few drops should be sprinkled upon a napkin and held an inch from the nose, allowing plenty of air to mix with its vapor. Ether may be confined in a cone and requires less mixture of air with its fumes. In case of threatened heart failure, lower the head until it touches the floor, and elevate the legs and body. Draw out the tongue with tongue forceps, an article that should always be at hand. Perform artificial respiration. Dilate the rectum. If no rectal speculum is at hand, insert two fingers of each hand, back to back, and stretch with all the force at command. We have found this new way very satisfactory. Hypodermic syringe loaded with brandy should always be at hand. Ammonia held to the nose or repeated slapping of the face with the end of a towel wrung out of cold water will tend to revive the patient. A patient is said to be under an anæsthetic when all rigidity of the limbs has ceased; the arm lifted up drops as a dead weight; the eye-lid can be raised without resistance and the finger can be pressed against the eye-ball without any signs of sensibility.

An **Ulcer** is any sore left by the destruction of the superficial parts of the skin or mucous membrane. A **Felon** or **Boil** is the result of some slight injury, as a scratch becoming infected with pus microbes. Incision should be made early. **Bed-sore,** or decubitus, is due to feeble circulation in some part that has been subjected to long continued pressure, as in cases of typhoid and other tedious diseases. Bed-sores are best prevented by washing suspicious spots with a solution of Tannic Acid. **Gangrene** is death of a part. There are two varieties. The moist and the dry The former is rapid in its progress, while the latter is slow and is commonly met in old age, in which case it is called **Senile Gangrene.** A suppuration of the tissues just beneath the skin is called a **Carbuncle.** It is commonly located on the back of the neck. A carbuncle is usually distinguished from a boil by the fact that it has more than one opening; often several.

A hypodermic injection of equal parts of Carbolic Acid and distilled water at a number of points in the circumference of the carbuncle, is highly recommended.

Shock is the impression made upon the nervous system by an injury. It varies from a transient sense of weakness to profound depression, with unconsciousness, or even death. The chief symptoms of shock are: Paleness and coldness of the skin; cold, clammy sweat on the forehead; rapid, feeble pulse; shallow, irregular respirations; a falling of the temperature below normal; usually, the patient lies with eye-lids half closed, conscious, yet paying no attention to what is going on around about him; the face is without expression; may be able to speak, but the mind is feeble; in the worst cases they may look on with a dreamy indifference, while their broken bones and crushed limbs are being dressed, with no sense of pain whatever.

Reaction from shock is indicated by a fuller and less frequent pulse, a more natural condition of the skin and return to consciousness. The shock from a surgical operation can be very much lessened by securing tranquility of mind and nerves before the operation, by a rest in bed a few days before, by operating in the morning and by keeping the body of the patient warm during the operation. Shock needs prompt treatment. If it occurs during a surgical operation, the operation must be suspended. The head, lowered. Bottles of hot water and warm blankets must be placed about the patient. Hypodermic injections of brandy should be given. **Camphor** is one of the best remedies for shock. Put a drop or two of the tincture upon the tongue. A hypodermic injection composed of equal parts of Brandy, Ether and Spirits of Camphor, is highly recommended. Death from shock may occur within a few minutes after the injury, or it may not for several hours.

To stop the **Hemorrhage** is the first requirement in treating a wound. Direct pressure upon the bleeding part will usually check it. A piece of folded linen will often answer temporarily. A stream of hot water, as hot as can be borne, directed upon the oozing surface, will check the bleeding from the smaller blood vessels. Iodoform gauze tends to check oozing. The larger vessels should be picked up and tied. If this cannot be done at once, tie a handkerchief or towel, with a knot in it, tightly about the limb or part, so as to bring pressure on the bleeding vessel. The treatment of hemorrhage, occuring with the various diseases, is given elsewhere; also, nose bleed.

Contusions are produced by blows from some hard, blunt object, or by a violent squeeze. Blood may be forced into the skin, giving it a black and blue appearance, but the skin is not broken. There is no open wound at the beginning. Contusions vary from a slight bruise to absolute crushing. The sooner the discoloration of the skin occurs the more superficial the injury.

Arnica and very hot water are useful in all contusions. A lotion composed of two drachms of Muriate of Ammonia and two ounces each of alcohol and water, is a very satisfactory application in both **Contusions** and **Sprains.** Apply by moistening a piece of thin gauze.

Burns and **Scalds** are essentially the same. They are classified according to their depth. Extensive burns, though superficial, are followed by profound shock. In fact, one-half of the fatal cases die from shock during the first forty-eight hours. A deep burn involving a small area of the surface is far less serious than an extensive superficial burn. In burns, the same care should be taken as in other wounds to prevent septic fever and suppuration. It is no more necessary that they should occur with burns than with other wounds.

The principle **treatment** of all burns is to protect the injured part from the air, prevent decomposition and make few changes of dressings. Blisters should be pricked, allowing the fluid to escape and the epidermis to return to its place. The pain from a burn may be relieved by washing with a solution of Bi-carbonate of Soda or a solution of Boric Acid. The latter is highly recommended. Powdered charcoal, bound over the burn, is said to relieve the pain and heal as if by magic. It is surely a good disinfectant. Burns of the throat from inhaling steam are relieved by inhaling the spray from an atomizer containing dilute Sulphuric Ether.

Camphor should not be forgotten in the shock from a burn. **Arnica** is useful in all cases. **Opium** may be necessary for children, to prevent convulsions following the great irritation of a burn.

Hernia, or rupture, is the escape of a part of the contents of a natural cavity of the body through a rent in its walls. The most common rupture is that met near the groin where the intestines sometimes escape through a rent in the abdominal wall. This form is called inguinal hernia. If it extends down into the scrotum, it is called scrotal hernia.

A carefully fitted truss should be worn. Hernia may be cured by injections of some astringent substance. The radical cure consists in cutting down and sewing up the rent. Even after this is done and healed up, it is necessary to wear a truss for a long time.

Fractures of bones are treated by placing the broken pieces as near as possible in their original position and maintaining them there by suitable splints and bandages for a period of three to six weeks. Splints made of Plaster of Paris, moulded to the parts, are very satisfactory.

Diseases of the bones and joints are frequently due to tuberculosis. The so-called white swelling or hip-joint disease is due to tuberculosis. The disease in the early stage in the joints may be cured by an injection of an emulsion of Iodoform and Glycerine. Ten per cent. of the former to 90 of the latter. Later stages of the disease require an operation for the removal of the diseased portions.

Homeopathy and **Surgery** go hand in hand. Many a case may be saved from the surgeon's knife by the indicated homeopathic remedy. Homeopathic treatment before and after a surgical operation will do much towards preventing complications and hastening recovery. The superiority of homeopathy in surgery has been demonstrated in the surgical wards of the Cook County Hospital, Chicago.

SECTION XV.

Mother and Child.

CONCEPTION.

Consists in the implantation of one of the microscopic germs, called spermatozoa, of the semen of the male in one of the eggs discharged from the female ovary. This implantation takes place somewhere within the womb or its appendages. Conception is most likely to occur immediately before or within the first two weeks after menstruation. The injuries done by the prevention of conception are discussed under the section, Diseases of Women.

PREGNANCY.

There are no positive signs of pregnancy before the fourth or fifth month after conception. There are many symptoms, however, that are strongly suspicious. First of all, the non-appearance of the menses. Yet the menses may cease from a number of causes. Morning sickness, consisting of nausea and vomiting in the morning, is another common symptom. It may be due occasionally to other causes. The pregnant woman, after vomiting, can eat again immediately, with relish.

Morning sickness usually continues from the beginning of the second month to that of the fourth. It may continue longer and be so troublesome that nothing can be retained in the stomach. Dirty, yellow blotches, called liver spots, often appear on the face during pregnancy. The breasts enlarge and the pink circles about the nipples become brown or black. The breathing has a peculiar labored character. No perceptible enlargement of the abdomen occurs until about the fourth month, or even later. The disposition undergoes a marked change. Sometimes, they are even peculiar and not unfrequently very irritable. Some enjoy the best health when pregnant, while others are miserable throughout. At the end of four and a half months, the mother usually, for the first time, feels the movements of the child in her abdomen. The date of confinement can be foretold quite acurately by counting forward four and a half months from the first time life is felt.

The best rule for the pregnant woman to observe is to be natural. Let her take plenty of exercise, without tiring; plenty of food, without over-eating; plenty of sleep, without becoming lazy. It is by far better that she have some congenial, active employment throughout pregnancy up to the hour of confinement. We have in mind a female physician, the mother of three children, who attended to her professional duties up to the hour of confinement, just as if she had not been pregnant. As a result of her great activity, she always had easy labors; never sick over an hour. It is a very great mistake for pregnant women to sit around with neither mental nor physical labor to do. Every muscle of the mind and body should be exercised daily in the open air. We say mind deliberately because the state of the mother's mind during pregnancy is reflected in the off-spring. A tendency to despondency, to murder, to steal, to drink, to fight, as well toward the high and noble, is often nothing more nor less than the imprint of the mother's mind while pregnant. Intercourse during pregnancy is believed to develop in the child a tendency to sensuality. Intercourse while nursing, sometimes affects the child badly.

Confinement is often preceded by a looseness of the bowels and a decided sinking of the abdomen. These occur about twenty-four hours before confinement. For days and even weeks before confinement there may be irregular pains here and there in the abdomen, called false labor pains. The real pains of labor come on at *regular* intervals. At first, perhaps half an hour apart. They gradually become more frequent until they occur every five minutes. They may be only three minutes apart. The physician should be present when the pains recur *regularly*, as often as every five or ten minutes. If the bowels have not moved freely just before the pains come on they should be evacuated by an injection of warm soap suds, to which has been added five drops of Carbolic Acid. The privates should be thoroughly bathed with soap and carbolized water. The room for confinement should be large, with plenty of ventilation, but no direct drafts.

It is very important that the heating facilities should be perfect. The mattress should be covered with a rubber sheet and over it again a clean linen sheet. The night-gown and shirt should be pinned above the waist and a clean sheet hung on a cord and the cord tied around the waist, so that the sheet answers in place of a skirt, and is the only covering below the waist. After delivery the cord about the waist is untied and the sheet, which is generally very much soiled, can then be easily removed. After which the unsoiled shirt and night-gown can be drawn down. If these precautions are not taken every article of clothing will be soiled and it will be necessary to change all the clothing of the patient; not any easy thing to do on account of the exhaustion.

Every woman is more or less injured or **torn** by the great stretching of the parts to allow the child to be delivered. The wounds p. juced should be dressed antiseptically, just as any other wound should be. Read the section previous to this one. A napkin of Iodoform gauze or Corrosive Sublimate gauze will be agreeable to the patient and do much toward preventing **child bed fever,** a disease that is rare wherever antiseptic precautions are used. An injection into the vagina up to the womb of a quart of warm water, to which there has been added ten drops of Carbolic Acid, is also a necessary precaution. It should be repeated daily; oftener, if there is any fever. Soon after labor, the abdomen sometimes becomes very **tender.** It should receive prompt treatment. It may be relieved quickly, as follows: Place by the bed a large kettle of boiling water. Lay over the abdomen a cloth rung out of Hamamelis. Over this apply dinner plates that have been dropped into the kettle of boiling water. Change the plates every three minutes for thirty minutes. If all soreness has not disappeared at the end of three hours use the plates again in the same manner for thirty minutes. In case, peritonitis occurs and the abdomen becomes distended, the temperature reaching 104 or more, apply to the abdomen a heavy bath towel wrung out of ice water. Reapply as often as it gets warm.

Retention of urine frequently occurs after delivery. For several hours there may be no desire or ability to urinate. After waiting a reasonable time, **Gelsemium** should be given. If this is not followed in due time by a passing of the urine, the catheter should be used to draw it. Immediately after delivery, it is customary to place a **bandage** around the abdomen. It is sometimes omitted without any bad results.

The **breasts** usually fill with milk on the third day. Its coming is often preceded by some discomfort, restlessness, elevation of temperature and headache; occasionally a slight, nervous chill. It should be remembered that fatal septicæmia may announce itself in almost the same way. Unless close observation is made, one may be mistaken for the other. We have known of more than one mistake of this kind. In septicæmia or child bed fever, the chill is usually pronounced and there is a sudden cessation of the flow. A stopping of the **flow** within the first three or four days should awaken alarm. If any soreness of the abdomen should occur with the stoppage of the flow, apply the hot plates as just described and give repeatedly injections of hot, carbolized water.

The rush of milk into the breasts may be so great as to produce enormous distention and pain. If not properly cared for at such a time, a **broken breast** may occur. Every woman who has had the misfortune to have one, will testify that they would rather have six children than one broken breast. We believe that a broken breast can always be prevented in the following simple manner: As soon as the breasts begin to be uncomfortable by the accumulation of milk in them, wrap the entire chest tightly with a bandage twenty yards long and three inches wide. Soft, white flannel makes the best bandage. Begin applying the bandage by wrapping it three times around the waist below the breasts and then three times under the arms above the breasts. Then carry it over the shoulder and back again around the waist and then over the other shoulder. Repeat until both breasts are covered and tightly bound down, with nothing but the nipples exposed. Within an hour after the bandage is put on, the milk should drain freely from both nipples. The bandage may be reapplied daily as long as necessary. Ointments, milk pumps and rubbing the breasts will be unnecessary. We have used the bandage for nine years and in hundreds of cases without a failure. The patient experiences immediate and great relief. We recall one severe case where the relief from the bandage was so great that the husband immediately presented us with the finest overcoat that could be made.

During the first four days after delivery, the mother should be kept perfectly quiet. She should not even raise her head from the pillow. The nurse should do it for her. All visitors should be kept out. The nurse should keep her own hands, person and clothes clean. They should be thoroughly disinfected before she assumes charge of the case. She should wash her hands often in carbolized water. The **diet** of the mother until after the third day should be simple and non-stimulating. No meat should be allowed during the first three days. The **Perineum**, the space between the front and back passage, may be ruptured down to the rectum, in cases where the head of the child is very large, or in cases improperly handled. It is best to sew up such tears immediately after delivery. It can be done quickly, with scarcely any pain. Every antiseptic precaution should be employed in performing this operation.

In case of profuse hemorrhage immediately after delivery of the child, *press* and rub *deep* over the abdomen until the womb is felt to contract into a hard ball, the size of a man's double fist and remains contracted. Take pillows from under the woman's head. Elevate the foot of the bed several inches. A chair will answer as a block or support in case of an emergency. A half teaspoonful of the fluid extract of Ergot may be given and repeated in ten minutes. A cord may be tied about one leg. **Ipecac** may also be given. Hemorrhage is often due to retention of a piece of the after birth. It is likely to persist until it is removed. An effective means of stopping sudden and profuse hemorrhage is for the physician to insert his hand, thoroughly cleansed, into the womb and scrape out with his fingers whatever remains that should come away. We have injected vinegar, successfully, in case of severe hemorrhage.

As soon as a woman learns that she is pregnant, it is well for her to put herself under the care of a good homeopathic physician and take such homeopathic remedies as may be from time to time indicated. **Arsenicum** is often indicated in morning sickness; also, after delivery when the flow is foul. It tends to prevent septic troubles; **Pulsatilla**, also. Claims are made that if this remedy is given during pregnancy it will facilitate the proper turning of the child in the womb, so that the head will be born first, as it should be, and not the feet or buttocks. **Sulphur** is also very useful for morning sickness; especially when there is vomiting at six o'clock in the evening. **Bryonia** is generally called for to increase the flow after confinement. **Belladonna** is often indicated in confinement cases

Abortion is the expulsion of the fœtus before the third month and **Miscarriage**, its expulsion between the third and seventh month. **Premature** labor is delivery between the seventh and ninth month. **Criminal** abortion is an abortion brought about intentionally. Criminal abortion is usually accomplished by drugs or by some instrument inserted into the mouth of the womb. There is nothing more ruinous to a woman's health, and very rightly, in most States, it is a penitentiary offense for a physician to induce an abortion. As a rule, half a dozen confinements will do less harm to a woman's health than one criminal abortion. A large proportion of the diseases of women date from abortion or miscarriage.

THE BABY.

After delivery, the baby's mouth should be cleared of everthing that may obstruct it. The cord should not be severed until all pulsations in it have ceased. This requires from five to twenty-five minutes. If the cord is cut before pulsation ceases, the child is more likely to be feeble and cross. Many testify to this peculiar fact and, it coincides with our own observations. The child may be simply oiled or washed and dressed. Great care should be taken that the child does not take cold by washing. It is better not to wash a feeble child until the next day. The eyes, however, should be cleansed in all cases. The child should be well wrapped up and laid on its right side in a warm place and *let alone*. It needs no food except what it can obtain from the mother's breasts. It should be put to the breast *regularly* every four hours. If absolute regularity is observed, it will make the child good and save the mother from many a sleepless night. To feed the child every time it cries is positively wrong and the most common cause of stomach trouble. No matter how much it cries, wait until the regular time to feed it. It may and should be given a teaspoonful of water when it cries persistently. Babies should be given plenty of water, especially in warm weather. During the first month, babies naturally sleep about twenty hours out of every twenty-four. In spite of the best care, they are sometimes colicky and cross during the first six weeks. It may be necessary to give them **Chamomilla, Colocynth, Ipecac** or some other internal remedy. But never give soothing syrups. They, as a rule, contain some injurious opiate. An infant's bowels should move from three to five times within twenty-four hours. A frothy, green stool indicates indigestion and colic. Constipation indicates insufficient nutrition. The mother's diet quickly affects the child. We recall a case, not at all unusual, where the mother ate cucumbers one day and buried her infant the next day as a direct result. Green vegetables, unripe fruits and ice cream are particularly liable to derange the digestion of the mother and seriously affect the child. The mother should not nurse the child after any strong emotions, as anger or fright. We recall a case where some of the plaster on the ceiling fell and frightened a young mother. The noise aroused the baby and she immediately nursed it. Within an hour or two, we were called, to see the baby on account of convulsions. Speaking of **Convulsions** reminds us that feeble health and convulsions in male children are very frequently due to a long foreskin. All male children should be examined early and, if necessary, circumcised. The old Jewish rite has much to commend it. While we have discussed convulsions in another section, we would repeat, that the best way to relieve a child in a convulsion is to strip it entirely and wrap it in a sheet wrung out of very warm water. Cold water will answer, if no warm water is at hand. About the sheet wrap a blanket. **Belladonna** is the usually indicated remedy in convulsions.

Every mother should nurse her baby whenever possible and, also, nurse it through the second summer. It must be remembered that, with the best care, the death rate among babies is very great, and that nothing increases an infant's chances of dying so much as to be deprived of its natural food, which its mother's breast alone can supply. A wet nurse is the best substitute for the mother. Cow's milk is the artificial food, generally used. In its natural state, it is too thick and contains too much cheesy matter. It also lacks milk sugar and readily becomes acid.

Great care should be taken to keep nursing bottles clean When not in use they should be soaked in water containing Bi-carbonate of Soda. The stopper is liable to become sour.

Milk may come from an unhealthy or improperly fed cow. It may be contaminated after it is drawn from the cow. For very young infants cow's milk should be diluted to one-third of its original strength with water and lime water. A teaspoonful of sugar of milk should be added to each bottleful of the mixture. There are many prepared foods on the market. It is well to give them in combination with milk. Condensed milk sometimes gives good satisfaction temporarily. It requires diluting to about one tenth. **Mercurius Sol** is one of the most useful remedies in case of stomach and bowel troubles of infants. It is indicated by a coated tongue. **Aconite** is useful for restlessness. **Belladonna** is very frequently indicated. Jerking and sudden crying call for it.

SECTION XVI.

Dietetics.

CLASSES OF FOOD.

Excepting air, water, minerals and fruits, every article of food belongs to one of three classes: The fats, the starches or the albuminoids. Butter is the best example of the fatty foods. It is almost pure fat. Rice, sago and potatoes are good examples of the starchy foods. The white of the egg and the lean of beef are examples of the albuminoids. An article of food may be made up of all classes, yet it is classified according to the one which predominates.

To prevent confusion of terms it should be remembered that the albuminoids are the albuminates, the proteids and the nitrogenous articles of food. While, the fats are the hydrocarbons and the starches the carbohydrates. An ideal diet should be made up from all three classes of food. The amounts of albuminoids and fats should be equal, while the amount of starches should be three times as great as either. Those of any class may take for a time the place of either of the others, but if long continued the body will not be well nourished. The amount of fats taken may vary more than either of the others. The seasons and temperature affect the quantity needed. The most constant requirement of the system is for the albuminoids or nitrogenous substances. Nitrogen is essential to all life. If lean meat alone be the diet, a large quantity will be needed to meet the wastes of the body. But if a small quantity of fat be added to the diet, the quantity of the lean meat or albuminoids needed will be much less.

The following articles are named in the order of the amount of **albuminoids** they contain. The percentage of each is also stated: Skim cheese, 44.8; cheese, 33.5; cooked lean beef, 27.6; peas, 23; white of egg, 20.4; raw lean beef, 19.3; raw lean mutton, 18.3; white fish, 18.1; veal, 16.5; yolk of egg, 16; entire egg, 14; oatmeal, 12.6; corn meal, 11.1; wheat flour, 10.8; fat pork, 9.8; rye meal, 8; rice, 6.3; buttermilk, 4 1; new milk, 4.1; skim milk, 4; cream, 2.7; potatoes, 2.1; cabbage, 2; butter and fats, 1;'beer, 1; arrow root and sugar, 0. Now, when we name these articles of food in the order of the amount of starch they contain there is a very great change. Arrow root, 82; rice, 79.1; rye meal, 69.5; barley meal, 69.4; wheat flour, 66.3; corn meal, 64.7; oatmeal, 58.4; peas, 55.4; potatoes, 18.8; parsnips, 9.6; carrots, 8.4; cabbage, 5.8; turnips, 5.1. If we name them in the order of the amount of fat they contain, there is still another change. Butter and fats, 83; dried bacon, 73; green bacon, 66.8; fat pork, 48.9; fat mutton, 31.1; cheddar cheese, 31.1; yolk of egg, 30.7; fat beef, 29.8; cream, 26.7; cheese, 24.3; tripe, 16.4; veal, 15.8; roast beef, 15.4; entire egg, 10.5; corn meal, 8.1; oatmeal, 5.6; barley, 3.9; new milk, 3.9; poultry, 3.8; white fish, 2.9; barley meal, 2.4; peas, 2.1; rice, 0.7; potatoes, 0.2; arrow root, 0. It will be noticed that arrow root has neither fat nor albumen, but contains 82 per cent. starch. It leads the list of the starches. Butter and fats have no starches and but one per cent. of albumen, but contain 83 per cent. fat and heads the list of fats. Skim cheese heads the list of the albuminoids. It contains no starch and but 6.3 per cent. of fat. After it, in the albuminoids follow ordinary cheese, roast beef, peas and white of egg. The white of egg is the purest example of albuminoid. It contains neither starch nor fat.

It will be noticed that dried peas are particularly rich in albuminoids and starch. The cereals are all rich in the starches. Corn meal contains more fat than any other cereal. Potatoes contain little besides starch. More than half of the body is water, 58.5 per cent. If the articles of food be named according to the amount of water they contain, they will appear as follows: Beer, 91; porter, 91; cabbage, 91; skim milk, 88; buttermilk, 88; new milk, 86; carrots, 83; turnips, 82; white of egg, 78; white fish, 78; salmon, 77; potatoes, 75; eels, 75; poultry, 74; entire egg, 74; ox liver, 74; lean beef, 72; lean mutton, 72; veal, 63; cream, 66; cooked lean beef, 54; fat mutton, 53; yolk of egg, 52; fat beef, 51; skim cheese, 44; fat pork, 39; ordinary cheese, 36.8; green bacon, 24; arrow root, 18; peas, 15; oatmeal, 15; rye meal, 15; wheat flour, 15; barley meal, 15; butter, 15; dried bacon, 15; corn meal, 14; rice, 13.

The following twelve elements enter into the composition of the human body: Carbon, hydrogen, oxygen, nitrogen, sulphur, phosphorus, chlorine, iodine, potassium, calcium, magnesium and iron. The first four in large quantities; the last eight, in small quantities. Food must contain all these elements. It is from this fact that the idea of the "twelve tissue remedies" was developed by Schussler. That is, disease is due to a lack of one or more of these elements and the cure consists in supplying the deficiency. All foods contain mineral salts. The following are the principal ones: Potash, soda, lime, magnesia, iron oxide, phosphoric acid, silicea. In naming the various foods according to the amount of mineral salts they contain, they will appear in the following order: Cheese, 5.4; lean beef, 5.1; skim cheese, 4.9; lean mutton, 4.8; veal, 4.7; fat beef, 4.4; fat mutton, 3.5; ox liver, 3; oatmeal, 3; dried bacon, 2.9; peas, 2.5; fat pork, 2.3; barley, 2; butter and fats, 2. Fruits consist almost entirely of water, sugar and mineral salts. Green vegetables are especially rich in salts, in proportion to the amount of solid matter they contain. A pound of fresh vegetables will contain, by weight, not more than one or two per cent. of salts, but if the large amount of water which they contain be extracted, they will form about ten per cent. of what remains.

By a few moment's study one can readily classify almost any article of food, and be able to form combinations that will make a diet that will nourish the body properly. In the combination of meat, bread and butter, we have all three classes of food. Thus, the meat contains the albuminoids; the bread, the starches, and the butter, the fat. If potatoes be added, it simply increases the amount of starch. It will be remembered that at least three times as much of the starches are needed as of the albuminoids or fats. A diet of oatmeal, eggs, beef and cheese would contain too much of the albuminoids. The system would soon rebel, showing itself, perhaps, in biliousness, if not in some more serious manner. Meat and eggs at the same meal would also make too much of the albuminoids. Eggs, potatoes and butter would be better. Cheese and potatoes represent all three classes of food. If macaroni, which contains 76.8 per cent. starch, should be added, the starches alone would be increased. A diet of arrow root, macaroni, crackers, potatoes and rice would be faulty, because all the articles belong to the starchy class. A diet of butter, cream, cheese, fat pork and smoked ham (36.5 per cent. fat) would also be faulty, because all the articles belong to the fatty class.

[The following table, abridged from Parkes, shows the composition of the chief articles of diet, and is also used for calculating diet tables. Figures of other authorities differ slightly:

Articles.	Water.	Proteids	Fats.	Carbo-hy'rates.	Salts.
Beefsteak.............	74.4	20.5	3.5	....	1.6
Fat pork...............	39.0	9.8	48.9	....	2.3
Smoked ham...........	27.8	24.8	36.5	....	10.1
White fish.............	78.0	18.1	2.9	....	1.0
Poultry................	74.0	21.0	3.8	....	1.2
White wheaten bread...	40.0	8.0	1.5	49.2	1.3
Wheat flour............	15.0	11.0	2.0	70.3	1.7
Biscuit	8.0	15.6	1.3	73.4	1.7
Rice	10.0	5.0	0.8	83.2	0.5
Oatmeal...............	15.0	12.6	5.6	63.0	3.0
Maize	13.5	10.0	6.7	64.5	1.4
Macaroni	13.1	9.0	0.3	76.8	0.8
Arrow root.............	15.4	0.8	....	83.3	0.27
Peas (dry).............	15.0	22.0	2.0	53.0	2.4
Potatoes...............	74.0	2.0	0.16	21.0	1.0
Carrots................	85.0	1.6	0.25	8.4	1.0
Cabbage...............	91.0	1.8	5.0	5.8	0.7
Butter	6.0	0.3	91.0	....	2.7
Egg (1-10 for shell)....	73.5	13.5	11.6	....	1.0
Cheese.................	36.8	33.5	24.3	....	5.4
Milk (sp. gr. 1032)......	86.8	4.0	3.7	4.2	0.7
Cream	66.0	2.7	26.7	2.8	1.8
Skimmed milk..........	88.0	4.0	1.8	5.4	0.8
Sugar	3.0	....	....	96.5	0.5]

The absolute amount of food required by an adult in twenty-four hours depends upon a number of conditions. The amount of each class of food is also dependent upon and varies according to different conditions. Every one knows that the fats produce heat and that not so much fat is needed in hot weather. As a general rule an adult engaged in *moderate* work requires every twenty-four hours, of fats, 3 ounces; of albuminoids, 5 ounces, and of starches, 14 ounces. At *rest*, of fats, 1 ounce; of albuminoids, 3 ounces, and of starches, 12 ounces. At *laborious* work, of fats, 3 ounces; of albuminoids, 7 ounces, and of starches, 18 ounces. The average amount of dry food needed is about 23 ounces. But food, as ordinarily eaten, contains from 50 to 60 per cent. water.

Some foods are more completely absorbed than others. For instance, sugar is completely absorbed, while the residue from gelatine is fifty per cent. It passes off as waste matter from the bowels. Animal food is more completely absorbed than vegetables. The residue from the latter being fully twice as great as that from the former.

Water is the most necessary article of food. Without water one can live but a few days. About three-fifths of the body is water. Pure water has no taste. Impure water is the chief if not the only source of such diseases as typhoid and cholera. The inorganic impurities may be removed from water by filtering. Germs may be killed by boiling the water for half an hour. A more effectual way of sterelizing water is simply to raise it three times to the boiling temperature and then let it cool after each time. Whenever typhoid or cholera, or any other bowel complaint prevails all drinking water should be boiled. Absolutely pure wa'er has great dissolving power. Gravel is often dissolved by it. There are numerous mineral waters on the market consisting of pure water, impregnated by nature with some mineral or minerals. Many are artificial. Mineral waters should not be drank unless specifically prescribed by a physician. Many springs in Europe have become famous for the cure of certain troubles. The specific therapeutical values of mineral springs of this country have not yet been determined. That Vichy water is of great value in case of a sour or irritable stomach, is a well established fact. A mineral iron water is believed to be also of value in Bright's disease. The value of hot water in case of chronic catarrh of the stomach, has been discussed in the section on diseases of the stomach.

Water should be drank when the stomach is empty. If drank while eating or after eating, digestion is disturbed. There is no drink that can take the place of pure water. Many persons do not drink enough water, while others drink too much. In certain nervous troubles, not enough water is drank, while in diabetes and Bright's disease, the craving for water is intense. The effects of taking large quantities of water is discussed under the head of Suralimentation.

Milk is the natural food of the young. This fact we learn from nature. A glance at the table on page 307 shows that it is nearly ninety per cent. water and contains all three classes of foods in nearly equal amounts. The large proportions of water and fat are well adapted to the needs of infants whose bodies it will be remembered are at least four-fifths water, but for adults, whose bodies it is estimated require 23 ounces of solid food every twenty-four hours, milk is not so good. It would require nine pints of milk to supply 23 ounces of solids. If one took nine pints of milk, he would take an excess of fats and of albuminoids. Bread added to milk increases the starch and makes the proportions of the three classes about what they should be for an ideal diet. Bread and milk is, therefore, a scientific as well as a palatable diet. A person, however, can live and do well for weeks on a diet exclusively of milk. In some diseases such a diet is necessary. Many persons have the erroneous idea that they cannot take milk; that it makes them bilious. Any person can take milk, if they start with small quantities; not more than six tablespoonsful at a time, beginning at 7 a. m. and repeating every hour and a half until 10 p. m. Three tablespoonsful given every hour and a half, from 7 a. m. to 10 p. m., makes a total of one pint. Six tablespoonsful at a time, equals one quart. Twelve, two quarts and eighteen, three quarts, all that is needed to nourish the patient. The patient may begin with three tablespoonsful and gradually increase the amount each day. Milk curdles at the beginning of digestion. If the curds are not dissolved again, they will be vomited up or evacuated from the bowels as curds. Carbonate of Magnesia or lime water or Vichy water added to the milk will prevent this difficulty. The taste of milk may be made palatable to those who dislike it, by boiling it with a stick of cinnamon. Milk should always be *sipped* and mixed with the saliva of the mouth. In this way, the heavy lump in the stomach felt by some will be avoided. Skim milk and buttermilk often agree when sweet milk does not. Kumyss is fermented milk made by adding yeast and sugar of milk to sweet milk. It contains about one per cent of alcohol. It is deservedly popular. Matzoon is a new preparation of milk resembling kumyss. We have never had milk in any other form satisfy our patients so well. They never grow tired of it.

Sweet cream diluted, sweetened and salted is a nutritious and palatable diet, often retained by very weak stomachs. Predigested milk, made by adding pepsin to raw milk and boiling, does well in some cases. It should always be kept in mind that milk is a food and not a beverage. It should never be taken simply to quench thirst. Milk readily becomes contaminated with germs and foul odors. Too great care cannot be taken to keep the milk vessels absolutely clean and covered, away from all impurities. The use of milk and hot water, to which salt has been added, is discussed under the head of diseases of the stomach. Many cases of long standing dyspepsia may be cured by an exclusive milk diet. The constipation that usually accompanies such a diet may be overcome by injections of water every other day or by taking liquorice powder. Milk is the ideal diet for Bright's disease. Many a case of insomnia, restlessness and bad dreams, along with indigestion and backache, may be readily overcome by an exclusive milk diet for a few days. Ninety-nine physicians out of a hundred use an exclusive milk diet in typhoid. We have our patients during the first week abstain from all food except water. During convalescence we give milk diluted, beginning with a very small quantity.

Flesh alone does not supply all the requirements of an ideal diet. One should not live on a purely meat diet. A glance at the table on page 307 shows that all meats are entirely lacking in the starches. They do, however, contain more or less fat, which may, in a way, take the place of starch. At this writing, the World's Fair Congress of Vegetarians is being held in Chicago. As a rule, vegetarians are simply non-meat eaters. The most of them eat eggs, butter, cheese, milk, nuts and fruits, as well as all the vegetables. Another glance at the table on page 307 shows us that it is no difficult matter to arrange a diet without meat, which will contain all three classes of food in proper proportions. The chief value of meat as a diet is the albuminoids; or, more properly speaking, the proteids, which they supply. Meat contains no starch and a variable amount of fat. But cheese contains more protein and more fat than the best beef steak. Peas contain almost as much of the proteids as meat, besides a very large amount of starch. But, it is a fact, that the proteids of meat are more readily digested than those of vegetables. This, perhaps, accounts for the fact that meat eaters get hungry sooner than vegetarians. The greater part of the human race are non-meat eaters. Some of the strongest nations physically eat little or no meat. Many notable examples of great age and activity might be cited among the vegetarians. It is claimed that cancer, consumption and other diseases are less prevalent among vegetarians. Whether this claim is true or not, we do not know. But our own observation convinces us that a meat diet, during an attack of an infectious disease, renders the disease more severe; or, in other words, it always has seemed to us that it made the germs of the disease thrive more vigorously. We do not know, however, but what any albuminous food might do the same. We are inclined to think that perhaps eggs, cheese or peas would aggravate an infectious fever just as much as meat does. Since writing the preceding, we notice that the eminent French physician, Dujardin-Beaumetz, says: "Food containing the least amount of albumen is best in fevers." According to our observation, feeding the patient "to keep his strength up" during a fever, is the best way to keep him *down*. We believe the germs are fed more than the patient. Albuminous or nitrogenous substances afford the most fertile soil for germs of disease. Nitrogen is an essential element to all life. There is no life where there is no nitrogen. The albuminoids or proteids alone contain nitrogen. It is not found in starch or fat. The albuminates are used to supply the waste of tissue and fluids of the body, especially the muscles, the nerves and the blood. Fat and starches both serve to save excessive waste of albumen. As already observed, a small quantity of fat added to lean meat lessens greatly the amount of lean meat needed. Fats economize the albuminates.

Fat enters into all the tissues. By its decomposition heat and force are produced. Both mental and muscular force. It is stored up in the body in greater or lesser quantities, in reserve, as it were, for emergencies. The amount of fat used and needed depends directly upon the amount of work performed. We have already observed that the amount of fat needed was more variable than either of the other classes of food. An animal fed on fat alone soon dies.

Starches do not enter into the tissues of the body, but are converted into other substances, contributing greatly to heat and mechanical force, also to an increase of the albuminoids and fats. If we desire to increase the muscular parts and not increase the fats, we must give an abundant of albuminates and little of the starches or carbohydrates. We have a practical example of this in the training of a prize fighter. He eats largely of lean meat and sparingly of vegetables.

Meat is mostly digested in the stomach and the starches in the intestines. In case of stomach derangement purely, meat is usually the first food the patient refuses. On account of the large percentage of meat digested and absorbed, the residue, is small. As a consequence the stools are smaller and less frequent where the diet is largely animal than it is when the diet is wholly vegetable.

Whether the vegetarian idea is correct or not, a diet largely of meat taxes the stomach and kidneys, and probably contributes to the development of rheumatism and gout. Meat once a day is a safe compromise. Oftener is too much for the average person. Meat three times a day is beastly in more senses than one. The value of meat is very much affected by the manner in which it is cooked. It should never be fried. In fact, no article of food should be fried. Meat should be cooked so as to retain the rich juices.

Cereals or grains are usually classed with the vegetables, but another glance at the table on page 307 shows us that they differ very widely from those we commonly think of as vegetables in the quantity of water they contain. For instance, rice contains but ten per cent. of water while potatoes contain seventy-four per cent. A person cannot live indefinitely on a cereal diet alone. Salisbury made the experiment of feeding four well and healthy men on an exclusive **oatmeal** diet for a month. The oatmeal was made palatable by being seasoned with salt, butter and pepper. Cold water was drank between meals and a pint of coffee, seasoned with sugar and milk, was taken at meals. Constipation, flatulency and colic soon developed, accompanied by dizziness, restless sleep, horrible dreams and weakness of legs. By the thirtieth day, each of them was having from eight to eleven evacuations from the bowels with all the other symptoms of a well established case of chronic diarrhœa. At the close of the thirtieth day, the oatmeal diet was suspended, a dose of Rochelle Salts given and a purely meat diet taken for the next four days, at the end of which time the men were well again. A study of the table again shows us that oatmeal alone as a diet contained a great excess of starch and that the bowels were unduly taxed, to digest it. He made a similar experiment on six strong, healthy men, with **baked beans**. They, too, soon developed symptoms of bowel trouble. By the tenth day each one developed symptoms of progressive paralysis or locomotor ataxia. By the sixteenth day, they dragged their legs and wobbled when they walked and could not raise their feet clear of the floor. By the nineteenth day, they were each having from ten to thirteen stools every twenty-four hours and, on account of the seriousness of their symptoms, the diet had to be suspended. Each one lost from nineteen to twenty-five pounds in weight. Beans are very rich in starches, but deficient in the fats and albuminates. The alarming symptoms developed in the men were produced simply by a diet that did not contain the three classes of food in proper proportion. It should be noted that these men also speedily recovered after a few days, on a diet exclusively of beef steak.

The same experiments were made with bread, rice, wheaten grits, hominy, sago, tapioca, potatoes, green peas, string beans, green corn, beets, turnips, squash, asparagus and the various meats. From four to six men were fed exclusively upon each one of these from seven to forty-five days. They could live upon any one exclusively of the first seven from forty to forty-five days before serious disturbances occurred. The diseased conditions that followed the exclusive use of each of the seven were very similar. Flatulence, weak heart, oppressed breathing, singing in ears, dizziness, headache, backache, constipation first, chronic diarrhœa afterwards, cold feet, numbness in extremities, general lassitude and weakness. Green peas ranked next to the first seven, but the exclusive use of either green corn, turnips, beets or squash, was soon followed by grave symptoms, Asparagus irritated the kidneys so that it was not safe to continue its exclusive use longer than seven days; after a few days the victim was scarcely able to walk. The experiments with meats showed that they, especially beef and mutton, can be lived upon exclusively, much longer without causing diseased conditions than the best vegetables. Cases are recorded where persons suffering from some grave disease have subsisted upon beef alone for years and become perfectly well. Eggs, fish, pork, veal, chicken, turkey and game may each, for a time, support life, but the continued and exclusive use of any one of them is likely to be followed by meat dyspepsia and scorbutic troubles. Meat dyspepsia is indicated by oppression and load about the stomach, with the sensation of a ball in the throat and the gulping of wind tasting like "rotten eggs."

These experiments, in the light of what we have already learned about diet, are sufficient to show us that the relation between diet and health are closer than is commonly supposed. Dietetics is a most important branch of knowledge that is not sufficiently studied or understood. Probably the origin of three-fourths of all diseases could be traced to errors of diet. Ignorance of hygienic cooking is universal. Poor cooks are injuring the health of the American people more than all other agencies combined. To be a good cook is really a fine accomplishment of which any woman should be proud, no matter what her station in life may be.

Fruits consist chiefly of sugar, salts and water. The fruit salts are very essential to perfect health. Fruit, in some form, should be eaten once every day. The best time to eat fruit is in the morning before breakfast, when the stomach is empty. If eaten when the stomach is full or before digestion is completed, they are likely to disagree or cause some disturbance of digestion. If eaten before breakfast, they will do more than physic to keep the bowels in a good condition. They will also soothe the nerves and sweeten the temper.

Rules. One should not eat when very tired, angry or excited. Rest before eating. Better sleep before eating a hearty meal than after. Drink before eating rather than during or after. Eat fruit when the stomach is empty. Do not continue long on one diet. Do not eat a great variety of food at one meal. Secure variety by eating different articles at different meals. Eat slowly and chew thoroughly. Be regular at meals. If faint between meals, drink a cup of hot water and take a dose of **Sulphur**. Coffee, tea and other stimulants are not necessary and often injurious. Do not "piece" between meals. It requires from two to five hours to digest most articles of food. If a new supply of food is taken into the stomach before it is empty, derangement is the natural result.

PART II.

Materia Medica.

THE DOSE AND PHARMACY.

The quality and not the quantity is the important feature in homeopathic medicines. A pound at a dose of any remedy may do more harm, but it can never do more good than a single grain. The smallest quantity of the indicated remedy, that is, the remedy which has indications exactly similar to the symptoms possessed by the patient, will be effectual, while a large amount of a remedy not indicated will have no effect; at least, no good effect. The quantity of the dose is, therefore, largely arbitrary. **Pellets** made from pure cane sugar are frequently used as a vehicle for homeopathic remedies. They are medicated by being saturated with the remedy in liquid form. The pellets are made in various sizes ranging from No. 8, the smallest, to No. 80, the largest. The number given to any size of pellet is determined by laying ten of equal size in a line and in close contact with each other; the length of the line given in millimeters is the number by which the particular size is designated. A number 30 pellet is about as large as a pigeon shot. It is the size commonly used. Five to ten of them, taken dry into the mouth, is a dose; five for children and ten for adults. The pellets may be dissolved in a part of a glass of water; in the proportion of two pellets to each teaspoonful of water. A teaspoonful of the liquid will, then, be the dose for children and a tablespoonful for adults. If the remedy to be used is in liquid form and not in a lower dilution than 2x, it may be mixed in water in the proportion of one drop for each teaspoonful of water. A teaspoonful of the mixture will be a dose for children and a tablespoonful for adults. If the remedy is in powder form, that is, in trituration, as it is commonly called, a quantity the size of a pea is the dose for children and the size of a large grain of corn for adults. A powder the size of two grains of corn may be put into half a glass of water. The dose, then, for children, would be one teaspoonful and for adults, one tablespoonful. Medicine thoroughly dissolved in water is more readily absorbed, less medicine is required and seems to act more satisfactorily. If the water is warm it acts still more quickly.

Crude drugs are generally diluted or attenuated several times before being used homeopathically. If the crude drug is in the form of a tincture, one part of it is mixed with nine parts of alcohol. The mixture is labeled 1x. One part of this mixture is also mixed with nine parts of alcohol and the second mixture thus formed is labeled 2x. One part of the 2x mixed with nine of alcohol makes the 3x. Higher dilutions are made in the same manner. One part of a given dilution mixed with nine parts of alcohol, makes the next higher dilution; 30x, 200x and even higher dilutions of some drugs are made and used with good results. If the crude drug is in the form of a powder or trituration, sugar of milk instead of alcohol, is used as the neutral vehicle by which the attenuation or thinning process is accomplished. One part of the powder of the crude drug is ground up or triturated with nine parts of sugar of milk to make the 1x trituration. One part of the 1x is triturated or ground with nine parts of sugar of milk to make the 2x. Higher potencies are made in a similar manner. The centesimal scale is sometimes used instead of the decimal. The proportions, then, are one part of the drug to ninety-nine of the neutral vehicle, the alcohol or sugar of milk, instead of one to nine, as in the decimal scale. The X mark following the number on the label indicates that the drug was prepared according to the decimal scale.

Remedies are usually given in potencies varying from 2x to 30x. Tinctures and potencies running up to the hundreds and thousands are occasionally given. The 3x and 6x, called the third and the sixth, are given almost universally.

The general rule is not to **repeat the dose** so long as there are signs of improvement. Most physicians, however, repeat the dose about every two hours in acute cases and every four or six hours in chronic cases. In case of emergency, as croup, convulsion or chill, doses may be repeated every ten minutes for four or six times and then less frequently, according to improvement. Some physicians, in cases of chronic troubles, repeat the dose of slow, deep acting remedies, such as Sulphur, Silicea, Sepia, Calcarea Carb, in high potencies, but once a day or once a week, or even but once a month. They claim splendid results. The great majority, however, repeat the dose three or four times a day.

The fundamental principle of homeopathy does not consist in the giving of small doses of diluted drugs, as many suppose, but in the giving to the sick person that drug which, if given in crude doses to a well person, produces symptoms similar to those possessed by the sick person. A collection of the symptoms produced by crude drugs upon healthy persons constitutes the **Homeopathic Materia Medica.** A definite symptom which is invariably produced in the well and as invariably cured in the sick by the same drug, may be called a **characteristic** indication of that remedy. Symptoms vary in their therapeutic value. General symptoms, such as "loss of appetite," "poor circulation," "fever," "headache," are too general and indefinite. Forty remedies may produce a headache. But a headache which begins at the nape of the neck and spreads over the top of the head, finally settling over the right eye, is definite and calls for **Sanguinaria.** It is the unusual and peculiar symptom that is of the greatest value in giving a clue to the indicated homeopathic remedy. In the succeeding pages, the leading characteristics are preceded by two dots, thus: ⁚. They have been repeatedly verified by hundreds and thousands of physicians and they may be relied upon with implicit confidence. Give but **one** remedy at a time. The remedies in parenthesis have symptoms similar to those they follow and should be compared. The remedies preceded by a star belong to the "twelve tissue remedies" of Schussler.

ACONITE.

⁚ Mental distress, fear, anxious, feverish, nervous, restless, (Ars., Rhus). Useful in the first stage of many troubles, after fright, injury, anger, chill, exposure to cold, dry wind. Skin, hot, dry, red, (Bell). Pulse, full, rapid, (Bell., Vera Vir.). ⁚ Sudden fever. Burning, pressing headache in forehead. Sensitive to light, noise, odors. Throat and windpipe sensitive. ⁚ Hoarse, dry cough, or croup cou...

ing on suddenly middle of night. Abdomen, hot, swollen and sensitive. Can't urinate. Tries often; passes drop, by drop. (Apis, Ars., Bell., Canth.) Stool, like chopped herbs. Bright hemorrhage. Numbness of left arm; also in legs after sitting. Cold feet. Ovaritis from taking cold during menses. Useful in acute inflammation in any part.

APIS.

Puffiness of skin or mucous membrane. Local dropsy. Stupor, interrupted by shrieks. Chronic meningitis. Absent-minded. Awkward. Eye-lids swollen, puffy, (Ars., Kali Carb). Baggy under eyes. Ears, nose, lips and face puffy. Waxy, pale. Inside of throat puffy, glossy red. Fever, without thirst, (Puls., Gels.). Bruised feeling in intestines. Anus feels raw. Stools pass with every motion of body, as if anus stood open. Stools, involuntary. Unconscious of stool. Right ovary enlarged, with pain in left side of chest. Suffocation. Sleepy. Intolerable, itching, stinging like bee sting. (Ars.) Trembling. Feeling as if toe or foot too large. Feet swollen, pale, waxy. Urine suppressed, or passed unconsciously. Frequent, painful urinations. Urine bloody or albuminous. Useful in **diphtheria**, Bright's, erysipelas, urticaria, cystitis, ovaritis.

ARNICA.

Bruised, sore feeling. First and most useful remedy in complaints from bruises, sprains, contusions, concussion. Strained eyes; over-exertion of any part. Mental as well as physical over-work. Whole body excessively sensitive. Dreads the slightest jar of the bed, (Bell.) Bed too hard. Head hot; body cold. Foul breath. Belching like rotten eggs.

ARSENICUM.

⁑ Anxious restlessness, (Acon., Rhus). ⁑ Rapid emaciation. ⁑ Worse after midnight. ⁑ Better by warmth. ⁑ Worse from drinking. ⁑ Drinks little and often. ⁑ Vomits as soon as food or drink reaches stomach. ⁑ Constant dread of death when alone or on going to bed. Face deathly pale, blue, dirty yellow. Features sunken and nose pinched. Cold sweat, (Veratrum Alb.), or dry skin with bran-like scurf. Eye-lids swollen, (Apis, Kali Carb). Watery diarrhœa, with vomiting, (Veratrum Alb.) ⁑ Burning in stomach, in anus, in eyes, in any part. Stools foul. Useful in any disease having any three of the foregoing symptoms. Useful in gastritis, ⁑ malaria, blood poisoning, asthma, cholera morbus, cholera, cancer, carbuncle, Bright's, epilepsy, anæmia, dropsy.

BAPTISIA.

⁑ Falls asleep while answering. Confusion of ideas. Muttering delirium. ⁑ Feels scattered into pieces. Can't go to sleep because he can't get himself together. Unable to think. Dull, bruised feeling in back part of the head. Face, dark red, besotted looking. Putrid sore throat. Can swallow liquids only. Abdomen, tender, especially right side. ⁑ Breath and all discharges foul. Drowsy, delirious stupor. Chilly all day. Whole body sore. (Arn.) Very useful in the beginning of typhoid and other troubles in which the blood is poisoned; diphtheria.

BELLADONNA.

▪ Flushed face, throbbing blood vessels, bounding pulse, wild delirium. ▪ Furious, bites, strikes and tears things, (Hyos., Stram.) Desires to escape. ▪ Intense, throbbing headache, worse by motion or noise. Violent throbbing. ▪ Shooting, stabbing pains. Pupils dilated. Can't bear light. Face, glowing, red and hot. Skin hot and moist. ▪ Throat dry, bright red and raw. Swallowing, difficult; feels constricted. Nausea. Dreads the slightest jar, (Arnica) Urine retained, passes drop by drop, (Acon., Apis, Ars., Canth., Nux). Pressing down. Feeling as if womb would fall out. Voice, husky, hoarse. Dry cough. Hoarse cry. ▪ Sleepy, but can't sleep. ▪ Smooth, bright scarlet redness of skin. Moans in sleep. Useful for sudden, violent fevers with great congestion; especially of the head. Chief remedy in scarlet fever, tonsillitis, congestive headache, delirium.

BRYONIA.

▪ All symptoms worse by motion. ▪ Stitching, tearing pains. Irritable temper. (Nux, Cham.). Depressed, (Puls.) Morning headache; pressing in forehead, in back of neck and down into the neck. ▪ Lips, mouth and tongue very dry (Ars.) Toothache better by cold water. All complaints better by lying on the painful side. Constipation. Stool, hard and dry. Coughs on entering a room. Stitches in chest on coughing or breathing, (Kali Carb). ▪ Joints red, swollen, stiff, painful on slightest motion. Nausea on sitting up. ▪ Dreams or talks in sleep about business. In delirium says he wants to go home. Useful in headache from indigestion, in rheumatism, meningitis, bronchitis, pneumonia, pleurisy, typhoid,

CACTUS.

! Sensation of a constriction about the heart, as if held in the grasp of an iron hand; as if it were squeezed; as if the heart had not room enough; as if cord around lower part of chest. Right sided headache and neuralgia. Congestion to head. As if would suffocate from constriction of throat. Hemorrhage of stomach, of lungs, of bladder, of bowels. Constriction of vagina. Oppression of chest. Attacks of suffocation. Sleepless. Intermittent fever without sweat. Paroxysms recur daily at same hour. Useful in heart disease, especially after rheumatism; angina pectoris.

CALCAREA CARB.

! Cold, clammy hands and feet. Swelling of glands of neck. Scrofulous, emaciated, but pot bellied. Backward in teething. Heat sweats while sleeping; sweats from slightest exertion. Toothache from slightest draft. Longing for eggs, chalk, slate, coal. Sour stomach after everything. Girls backward in menstruating. Menses return from least excitement; too profuse or two scanty. Leucorrhœa. Bone diseases. Tuberculosis or so-called white swelling of joints. Dizzy and out of breath going up but a short flight of stairs. Useful in all cases of poor nutrition. Headache of school girls. Results from sexual abuse.

CAMPHOR.

! First remedy in cholera or cholera like symptoms. Cold, clammy sweat, with vomiting. (Veratrum Alb.) Icy cold all over. Nose pinched and cold; tongue, cold; breath, cold; limbs, cold.

Very useful in shock. Pulse, very weak or not perceptible. First remedy when taking cold. Feeling as if cold air were blowing over covered parts. Excessive sexual desire in females. Cramps in calves. In suppressed eruptions, especially of measles. Urination, painful.

CHAMOMILLA.

⁞ Excessive sensitiveness. ⁞ Peevish, iritable. (Nux). Snapish. Dislikes to be spoken to. Useful during teething. Child quiet only when carried. Wants everything. Refuses everything. Convulsion from teething, anger, stomach or bowel irritation. Soothes the excitable. "The Opium of homeopathy." Stools green, watery, slimy, foul, like chopped egg and spinach. Colic. Sleepless. (Bell.) One cheek red. Violent, rheumatic pains.

CHINA.

⁞ Excessive sensitiveness of the nervous system. ⁞ All symptoms aggravated by touch, motion, physical or mental effort. Weakness following great loss of blood, semen or after diarrhœa or prolonged nursing. Profuse sweat. Lacks energy. Dullness, Skin and eyes yellow. Bloody leucorrhœa. Throbbing headache. (Bell.) Aching in back part of head after sexual excess. Scalp, sensitive. Roaring in ears. Pupils dilated. Belching. Dyspepsia. Impotence. No hunger, no thirst. Can't loose sleep.

CINA.

⁞ Picking of the nose. ⁞ White and bluish about mouth. ⁞ Sickly blue rings about eyes. Hungry soon after eating. The worm emedy. Worm spasms. Grinding of teeth while asleep. Constipation of children. Child wakens frightened. Pitiful weeping. Irritable. (Cham., Nux, Bry.) Wants everything. Urine milky.

COLOCYNTHIS.

Severe, colicky pains, obliging patient to bend double. Terrible, twisting, drawing, griping, cutting pain about the naval. Colic so severe presses abdomen against something hard for relief. Feeling as if intestines were being squeezed between stones. Colic from eating fruit or from drinking cold water when over-heated. Cutting in abdomen as if from knives. Vomiting and diarrhœa from anger. Painful menstruation. Stitches in the ovaries. Suppression of menses from chagrin. Bitter taste. (Acon.) Useful in neuralgia of any part. Especially sciatica. Bloody, mucous stools after eating. Glaucoma.

DIGITALIS.

Extremely slow, intermittent pulse. Faints; cold sweats; deathly look; Bluish lips. Deathly nausea. Dropsy; distending abdomen with suppression of urine. Nightly emissions. Menses suppressed, with hemorrhage from lungs. Sensation as if heart stood still. Pulse, feeble, irregular; sometimes violent. Valvular disease. Fingers "go to sleep." Weakness of left arm. Skin, eye-lids, tongue, lips and nails blue.

GELSEMIUM.

Fever without restlessness, Drowsy, languid and quiet. Opposite of Aconite. Trembling and weak. Complete relaxation; mental and muscular prostration. Limbs give out from least exertion. Feeling as if heart would stop unless one kept moving. Opposite of Digitalis. Dizzy; staggers; vision blurred, or double. Eye-lids droop. Tongue, numb and thick. Tingling here and there Diarrhœa after excitement. Sexual weakness; emissions upon slight provocation. Nervous chill. Paralysis following diphtheria. Bladder, weak. Pulse, weak, slow. Often useful in first stage of catarrhal, eruptive, bilious, remittent and typhoid fever. Neuralgia with menstruation; meningitis; convulsions; pain in neck; fever without thirst. (Puls., Apis).

GRAPHITES.

: Moist, sticky, scabby eruption; moist, itching eczema, with a honey-like fluid; massive, dirty crusts on head, matting the hair; painful and sore to touch; moist and raw behind ears; bleeding cracks behind ears, corner of eyes, nose, mouth, about nipples, anus, or in skin of hands. Lids red and margins scurfy. Ulceration of cornea. Pustules on cornea and conjunctiva. Catarrhal deafness; hears better amid noises. Smell acute; nostrils sore and blocked with dried, foul scabs. Constant sensation of cobweb on face. Sickening, rotten taste mornings; burning blisters on tongue; aversion to meats and sweets. Eruptions and ailments from suppressed menses; acrid leucorrhœa. Sad, tearful, (Puls.); music brings tears; fidgety; apprehensive; thick nails; herpes zoster; cancer of breast and womb; removes scabs; obesity.

HEPAR SULPHUR.

: Tendency to maturate. : Every little injury of skin suppurates. Scabs, itch and easily torn off, leaving a raw, bleeding surface. Ulcers, sensitive, bleeding easily; foul, corroding discharge.

Constant foul odor from body. Sweats easily. (Calc. Carb, China, Phos.) Unhealthy skin. Violent itching. Conjunctivitis, with much pus. Pimples and pustules around ulcers. Sensation of splinter sticking in throat. Desires vinegar. Tonsillitis. Croup. (Acon., Spong.) Croupy cough. Bronchitis. Abscess in any part. Hastens or arrests suppuration.

KALI BICHROMICUM.

■ Excessive secretion of sticky, tough, stringy mucus; acts upon the mucous membrane of eyes, ears, nose, throat, bronchi, stomach, rectum, kidney and liver, producing catarrh, erosion and often ulceration. Ulceration of eyes and ears. Nose dry, ulcerated, foul, filled with clinkers of tough, green plugs. Syphilis of mouth. Hawks tough, stringy mucus mornings. Diphtheria. Diphtheritic or membraneous croup. Pearly deposit. Hoarse cough; hoarse; voice gives out; difficult breathing; wheezing; dyspepsia; catarrh or ulceration of stomach. Nausea and vomiting of drunkards. Diarrhœa, brown, frothy; expectorations so tough strings out to the floor. Neuralgia every day at same hour. Deep, yellow ulcers.

LYCOPODIUM.

■ Full of gas. ■ Hungry, but loses appetite after first mouthful. Excessive appetite. More eaten, more craved. Hungry after eating. ■ Wakes in the night hungry. ■ All symptoms worse at 4 p. m.; better at 8 p. m. ■ Red sand in the urine. Rectum contracted, causing chronic constipation. Weeps. (Puls., Graph.) Sensitive spirit. Ailments from fright, vexation or chagrin. Throbbing headache. (Bell., China). Hair falls out. Eyes inflamed and stuck together; can't endure light; sees spots. Styes, granulated lids. Oozing behind ears. (Graph.) Nose obstructed; thick, yellow discharge. Snuffles. Fan-like motion of nostrils. Complexion muddy, pimply. Ulcers in mouth. Feeling of a ball rising in throat. Enlarged tonsils. Everything tastes sour. Pit of stomach sensitive. Rumbling in left side of abdomen. Coughing hurts abdomen. Violent colic from passing stone from gall bladder or kidney. Dropsy. Anus raw. Sexually weak. One foot hot. Expectorates small, greenish, yellow masses. Pneumonia. Enlarged veins on legs. Numbness. Gouty. Sweat immediately after chill. Diphtheria beginning on right side.

MERCURIUS SOL. (Viv.)

All symptoms worse at night and from the warmth of the bed. Worse when sweating. The effects of mercurial and syphilitic poisoning are almost exactly similar. Tongue coated, showing impress of teeth. Stools bloody and slimy, with much straining. Dysentery. Feeling of iron hoop about head. Syphilitic eye troubles. Vision dim. Foul, bloody discharge from any part. Inflamed glands. Teeth, loose. Gums, spongy, bleed easily. Throat, dry. Saliva, profuse. Frequent urging to urinate. (Canth., Apis, Bell.) Foreskin, sore. Privates, raw and itch. Breath, foul. Night sweats. Skin and whites of eyes yellow. **Mercurius Cor.** Discharges, corrosive, burn. Violent inflammations of mucous membrane. Burning in eyes, throat, bladder, rectum. Acute Bright's. Albuminous urine. Cystitis. Dysentery. Great straining when bowels move or urine pass. Scrofulous, gonorrhœal or syphilitic inflammation of eyes. **Mercurius Iodide,** called Yellow Iodide, acts especially upon the glands of the throat. **Biniodide of Mercury,** called Red Iodide, is useful in throat troubles; worse on the left side.

NUX VOM.

Bad effects from continued errors of diet, irregular or sedentary habits, highly seasoned food, stimulating drinks, strong drugs, mental strain, sexual excess and dissipation in general. Ill-humored, (Cham.) Inclined to swear. Head feels too large; confused, as if had not slept well. Nose runs all day; stops at night. Snuffles. No appetite. Nausea. Dyspepsia, from worry and study. Bilious. Desire to move bowels, but can't. Piles. Urine dribbles. Emissions. Falling of womb. Morning sickness. Rawness in chest. Lumbago. Unsteady gait. Convulsions. Trembles. Awakens at 3 a. m. Thinks much for an hour. Falls asleep. Wakens late more tired than on retiring. Load in stomach.

PHOSPHORUS.

Small wounds bleed much. Mucous membrane pale. Tall, slender, nervous blondes often need it. Emaciation. (Ars.) No mental or physical energy. (China) Gloomy. Chronic meningitis. Softening of brain. Dandruff. Sparks before eyes on trying to go to sleep. Blows blood from nose. Nose swollen. Mouth bleeds. Cotton sensation in throat. Palate, elongated. Thirst for cold drinks or something juicy. Vomits blood. Empty, faint feeling in stomach. (Sulp.) Profuse, painless diarrhœa. Chronic constipation. Stool, cigarette size. Piles. Impotent, yet desire great. Lascivious. Weakness from excess. Windpipe painful. Oppressed breathing. Congestion and heaviness of chest. Crackling in lungs; beginning of tuberculosis. Feet, icy cold. Locomotor axtia. Night sweat. (China, Calc.) Useful during convalescence from many diseases. Bluish hue. Fatty degeneration. Anæmia. Chlorosis. Purpura hemorrhagica.

PULSATILLA.

"Blues." Homesick. Cries easily; tears flow at the mention of her symptoms. Feels better out-doors. Can't breathe indoors. Turns up nose at the mention of fat meat. Fever without thirst. (Apis, Gels.) Headache from eating pastry or fat. Evening headache. Styes. Catarrh of eyes, ears, nose, throat. Painless leucorrhœa. Suppressed menses. Suppressed gonorrhœa with swollen testicle. Mumps. All discharges, bland, thick, yellowish or greenish. Rumbling in bowels (Lyc.). Night diarrhœa. Menstrual colic. Measles. Snuffles. Chlorosis, which iron has failed to cure. Wandering rheumatism. Inflamed veins.

RHUS TOX.

Better by motion. Opposite of Bryonia. Restless. (Acon.) Feels comfortable in each new position only for a few minutes. Effects of getting wet while over-heated; over-exertion. Muscular rheumatism following getting hands or feet cold or wet. Left sided troubles. Can't remain in bed at night; must walk about; can't sit still. Inflamed eyes. Mumps. Erysipelas spreading from left to right; dark colored; burning, itching eruption; eczema; raw surface; thick crusts; offensive oozing. Hives from getting wet. Typhoid when bowels are loose. Pains, as if flesh were torn from bones. Soreness and stiffness of muscles. Eruption of painful white vesicles. Worse before a storm.

SULPHUR.

▌Weak, empty, hungry, faint feeling in the stomach about 11 a. m. ▌Top of head hot. Rumbling and gurgling in bowels. (Lyco., Puls.) Painless diarrhœa, driving patient out of bed at 5 a. m. ▌Soles of feet hot; must uncover them at night or place them against a cool surface. Rush of blood to head. Feels too warm; wants doors and windows open, (Puls.) Chronic diarrhœa. Prevents cholera. May be useful in any disease, as sulphur enters every particle of protoplasm. The king of skin remedies. Itching piles. Hot flushes. All discharges, acrid and burn. Walks stooping. ▌Offensive odor from body, notwithstanding frequent washing. Itching all over. Skin rough, dirty, scabby. Fetid sweat about privates. ▌Lips very bright red. Painful smarting of eyes. Eyes blur. Itching pimples. Children dread being washed. Foolish pride over trifles. Sweat of arm pits stains clothing red.

MINOR REMEDIES.

Abies Nigra. Sensation of an undigested, hard-boiled egg in the stomach. **Abrotanum.** Marasmus of children. **Æsculus.** Severe aching pain across hips. Piles, protruding and purple. Ineffectual urging to stool; rectum feels as if full of sticks; back gives out when walking. **Æthusa.** Child can't take milk; passes it in curds, or vomits *forcibly* and falls asleep. **Agaricus.** Burning, shooting pains in spine, sensitive to touch. **Agnus Castus.** Premature decline of sexual power. **Ailanthus.** Purplish appearance in malignant scarlet fever. **Allium Cepa.** Acute catarrh with profuse, bland secretion from eyes and nose. **Aloes.** Diarrhœa; hastens to stool after eating; passes without exertion; fæces and urine escape together. **Alumina.** Rectum seems too dry; constipation of nursing infants. **Ammonium Carb.** Malignant scarlet fever, with much swelling of throat and stupor. **Ammonium Mur.** Fæces covered with mucus. Cold between shoulders; catarrh of chest. **Anacardium.** Brain fag; insanity; inclined to swear; sensation of a *plug* or band; suspicious; loss of memory. **Antimonium Crud.** Thick, milky, white coating on tongue; fretful, sulky. **Antimonium Tartar,** or tartar emetic. Rattling of mucus in the chest, with vomiting and drowsiness; pneumonia; bronchitis; small pox; pustules; debility; cold sweat; suffocation; new born infants purple; whooping cough. **Apocynum.** Dropsy. Use teaspoonful doses of tincture, **Argentum Met.** Chronic hoarseness; laughing provokes cough; expectoration like boiled starch. **Argentum Nit,** Mucus and pus mixed in all discharges from the part of the mucous membrane affected; ophthalmia; gonorrhœa; catarrh of stomach; dysentery; corners of eyes look like pieces of raw meat; green stool; sensation of splinter in throat; spinal irritation; epilepsy; brain fag, with irritability and trembling; melancholia. **Arsenicum Iodide.** Consumption and other debilitating diseases; night sweats; eczema; psoriasis. **Arum Triphyllum.** Discharges from nose makes the skin raw wherever it touches; corners of mouth cracked and bleeding; diphtheria and malignant scarlet fever. **Asafœtida** Sensation of ball rising in throat; hysteria. **Aurum.** Third stages of syphilis; suicidal tendency; fatty degeneration of the heart, liver, kidneys.

Baryta Carb. Enlarged tonsils; fatty tumors; aneurism. **Benzoic Acid.** Odor of urine exceedingly strong, offensive, pungent. **Berberis.** Sticking, digging, tearing, throbbing pain in region of kidney, extending to bladder and urethra; back stiff and lame; rises with difficulty. **Bismuth.** Terrible neuralgia of stomach; pain extends to spine; temporarily relieved by cold drink. **Borax.** Dread of downward motion; sore mouth and diarrhœa of infants; leucorrhœa like white of egg. **Bromium.** Croup; hoarse; loss of voice; paroxysms of suffocation; every inspiration excites cough; sudden choking.

* **Calcarea Flourica.** Enlarged blood vessels; piles; blood tumors; aneurism; bony tumors. * **Calcarea Phos.** Tonic during convalescence; chlorosis; anæmia; craves bacon; night sweats; teething, slow; scrofulous; Pott's disease; school girl headache **Calcarea Iodide.** Cures fibroid tumors. * **Calcarea Sulp.** Useful wherever there is pus. **Cannabis Indica.** Gonorrhœa with chordee, or painful erections. **Cannabis Sativa.** Terrible burning and smarting in urethra; worse after urinating. **Cantharis.** Constant urging to urinate, scanty discharge and violent, cutting, burning pains in urethra before, during and after urinating. **Capsicum.** Terrible burning and straining on urinating or moving bowels. **Carbo Animalis.** Cancer of womb or breast; old, foul ulcers; acne; dyspepsia. **Carbo Veg.** Full of gas; body cold; skin blue; breath cold; belches; colic; hemorrhages; collapse of exhausting diseases. **Caulophyllum.** Rheumatism of small joints; labor pains too weak. **Causticum.** Loss of voice; urine passes on coughing or sneezing; paralyses about face. **Cedron.** Symptoms return with clock-like regularity. **Chelidonium** Constant pain under right shoulder blade; liver remedy. **Cicuta.**

Convulsions with terrible contortions. **Cimicifuga.** Rheumatic, neuralgiac, choreic affections in hysterical women, arising from womb; painful menses. **Clematis.** Swollen testicle after suppression of gonorrhœa. **Cocculus.** Sea sickness; dizzy, as if intoxicated; paralytic tendency. **Coccus Cacti.** Laryngitis, bronchitis and whooping cough. **Coffea.** Morbid acuteness of all the special senses; excessive nervous excitability; sleeplessness. **Colchicum.** Tearing pains; terribly worse at night; gout; rheumatism; weak. **Collinsonia.** Piles, with heart trouble. **Conium.** Old persons; hardened glands; enlarged prostate; cancer; cough on lying down; dizzy on turning over; results of continence. **Corallium.** Whooping cough. **Crocus.** Hemorrhages, black; jumping sensation inside. **Crotalus.** Yellow fever; blood poisoning. **Croton tig.** Diarrhœa *forcibly* shoots out of the rectum; eczema. **Cuprum.** Convulsions; cramps in cholera; whooping cough; epilepsy.

Dioscorea Bilious colic; must stretch out; **opposite of** Colocynth. **Drosera.** Hoarse, spasmodic cough; whooping. **Dulcamara.** All symptoms worse in cold, damp weather; catarrh; rheumatism. **Eucalyptus.** Malarial fevers. **Eupatorium Perf.** Aching and soreness in muscles; violent bone pains; vomits bile after chill; malaria.

Ferrum. Anæmia; green complexion; chlorosis; better by gentle motion. * **Ferrum Phos.** Resembles Aconite and Rhus. Useful remedy in sudden fever of children.

Glonoin. Throbbing in brain; congestion; arteries stand out on temples; face pale; sunstroke; angina pectoris; apoplexy; insanity. **Hamamelis.** Dark hemorrhage; enlarged veins. **Helleborus.** Water on the brain; rolls head; boring into pillow. **Helonias.** Weak, tired, dragging, aching, burning across back and hips. **Hydrastis.** Weak, faint; catarrh with ropy discharge; erosion. **Hyoscyamus.** Acute mania and delirium occuring during other diseases; typhoid; illusions; hallucinations; sleepless; night cough. **Hypericum.** Useful after injuries of spine or nerves of hands or feet. **Ignatia.** Silent grief; sighs; now laughing, then crying; changeable; hysterical. **Iodium.** Emaciated, but hungry; scrofulous; croup; goitre. **Ipecac.** Persistent nausea and vomiting; stool, green as grass; hemorrhage of womb. **Iris.** Burning from mouth to anus. **Kali Carb.** Sticking pains; upper lids puffy; coughs at 3 a. m.; anæmia; prevents miscarriage; backache. **Kali Iodide.** Resembles mercury; antidotes mercury; syphilis; scrofula; rheumatism. *__Kali Mur.__ Resembles Bell. Thick, white discharges. * **Kali Phos.** Brain fag; insomnia. Useful for convalescents. *__Kali Sulp.__ Thin, bright, yellow or greenish discharges. **Kalmia.** Rheumatism of heart; slow, weak pulse. **Kreosotum.** Acrid, foul discharges; burning leucorrhœa; consumption; cancer; carbuncle. **Lachesis.** All symptoms worse after sleep; throat sensitive externally; left sided sore throat; diphtheria; blood poisoning. **Ledum.** Rheumatism of smaller joints; punctured wounds; sting of insects; violent itching. **Leptandra.** Tar black stool; bilious. **Lilium Tigrinum.** Bearing down as if womb would fall out; palpitation; leucorrhœa. **Lithium.** Rheumatism of heart with eye trouble; gout; small joints. **Lycopodus.** A substitute for Digitalis. **Magnesia Carb.** Stools green, frothy, like frog pond scum; acid dyspepsia. * **Magnesia Phos.** Sharp, cutting pains; colic; spasms. **Mezerum.** Syphilis and scrofula; after abuse of mercury. **Millefolium.** Bright red hemorrhage from lungs. **Muriatic Acid.** Great debility in long lasting fevers. *****Natrum Mur.** Long lasting, badly treated cases of malaria; chill every other day at 11 a. m.; craves salt; finger nails get blue. *****Natrum Phos.** Acid dyspepsia; sour vomiting. *****Natrum Sulp.** Liver troubles; uric acid. **Nitric Acid.** Syphilis after abuse of mercury; bleeding ulcers. **Nux Moschata.** Drowsiness; hysteria. **Opium.** Fright; constipation; epilepsy; stupor; snoring respirations; blue face. **Oxalic Acid.** Softening of spine. **Petroleum.** Eczema; herpes; ulcers; sea sickness. **Phosphoric Acid.** Mental dullness; physically weak; homesick; disappointed love; spermatorrhœa. **Physostigma.** Contracted pupils; tetanus; chorea; ataxia; paralysis of the insane. **Phytolacca.** Syphilitic and gonorrhoeal rheumatism; resembles Mercury and Kali Iodide; lumps in breast; reduces fat. **Picric Acid.** Brain fag; neurasthenia; great prostration. **Platina.** Mental and womb trouble combined. **Plumbum.** Neuralgia; sciatica; paralyses of legs. **Podophyllum.** Bilious troubles; painless morning diarrhoea; jaundice. **Rhododendron.** All symptoms worse before a storm, or by cold and dampness. **Ruta.** Bruises of bones and sprains. **Sabina.** Hemorrhage of womb. **Sanguinaria.** *Cures Polypi;* sick headache; bronchial troubles. **Secale.** Hemorrhage of womb or bowel; gangrene; fibroid tumor. **Sepia.** Displacement of womb; bearing down sensation; yellow blotches on face; bilious; palpitation. *****Silicea.** Long lasting suppurations; abscesses; ulcers; felons; boils; carbuncles; bone decay; scrofula. **Spigelia.** Facial neuralgia; spreads from one point; rheumatic eye trouble; symptoms rise and decline with the sun. **Spongia.** Croup; dry, wheezing sawing respiration; suffocation. **Stannum.** Lung trouble, with much expectoration of balls of sweetish mucus; chest weak. **Staphisagria.** Scrofula of glands and bones; styes; decayed teeth; sexual excesses. **Stillingia.** Secondary and tertiary syphilis. **Stramonium.** Delirium and acute mania; hallucinations of terrible things; incessant talking; hydrophobia. **Terebinthina.** Suppression of urine; blood and albumen in urine. **Teucrium.** Polypi. **Thuya.** Warts about anus following gonorrhoea; bad effects of vaccination. **Trillium.** Hemorrhage of womb. **Ustilago.** Hemorrhages from fibroid tumors of womb. **Valerian.** Hysteria; insomnia. **Veratrum Alb.** Cholera like conditions; cold sweat on forehead; terrible colic; cramps in calves; violent, watery vomiting and purging; feeble pulse. **Veratrum Viride.** Intense congestion of brain and lungs; very high temperature; rapid, full, strong pulse; pneumonia; meningitis; sunstroke; insanity. **Viburnum Opulus.** Painful menstruation; very useful. **Zincum.** Exhaustion of brain and spinal cord; brain fag; chronic headache and neuralgia; fidgety feet.

APPENDIX.

Homeopathy Explained.

The word homeopathy is derived from two Greek words, *homoios* and *pathos;* the former meaning *like* and the latter *pain.* The cardinal principle or fundamental law of homeopathy is expressed by the Latin phrase *"Similia similibus curantur."* It is liberally translated "Like things are cured by like." This idea had been hinted at by medical philosophers for ages, but it was left for a very learned physician in his day, Samuel Hahnemann, born in Germany 1755 and died in 1843, to make a practical application of the theory. He is, therefore, called the founder of the system of medicine known as homeopathy, and which has grown in popularity in almost a geometrical ratio for nearly a century.

The theory of homeopathy is *to give to the sick person that drug which given to a well person will produce in the well person symptoms similar to those possessed by the sick person.*

Any drug given in frequently repeated, large, strong doses to a well person for any considerable time, will produce in that person conditions or symptoms not previously possessed and always deviations in a greater or lesser degree from perfect health. Different drugs will produce different symptoms. No two drugs produce exactly the same set of symptoms. One will act mostly upon one part, while another acts upon another part.

Experimenting upon healthy persons to determine what effect a drug will have is termed the *proving* of the drug.

Hahnemann was a persistent toiler, a systematic student, a close observer and a profound thinker. Even outside of medicine he was recognized as a scholar, being an authority in chemistry and some of the allied branches. While translating a standard medical work of his day he noticed that Peruvian bark produced in healthy persons symptoms similar to those which were cured by it in the sick. He thus became impressed with the idea which he afterward named homeopathy. He made numerous provings upon himself, and upon others, of all the principal drugs known in his day. He carefully noted and classified all symptoms that could be attributed to the action of a given drug. The great majority of his observations have stood the test of time and will continue to be true for ages to come.

He and his followers have learned much from cases of accidental poisoning by various drugs taken internally.

His large collection of symptoms was the beginning of the homeopathic materia medica. It has been added to until now the complete homeopathic materia medica if brought into one work would be as large as one of the great encyclopœdias, and would include a description of the physiological action—that is, their action upon well persons—perhaps of a thousand drugs.

For instance, it was commonly observed that after a number of well persons had taken Belladonna, each one had a peculiar throbbing headache with stabbing pain from temple to temple. A wild, violent, active delirium was also noticed in many who had taken Belladonna. As a rule the skin became scarlet red, the throat dry, raw and also of an intense bright redness. The eyes were staring, projecting and sparkling. The silly custom among weak-minded girls of putting Belladonna into their eyes to make them sparkle is well known. The physiological action of Belladonna having been determined by experiments upon the healthy, it was an easy matter, according to the theory, that "like cures like," to determine in what sick conditions Belladonna would be useful. In case of scarlet fever where the skin was bright red, the throat dry, red and raw, the temples throbbing with pain and the eyes sparkling, along with delirium, we would have an excellent picture of Belladonna. The most stupid observer could not fail to notice the similarity between the symptoms produced by Belladonna upon a well person and those exhibited by the person sick with scarlet fever. If, after taking Belladonna, all the symptoms of the scarlet fever patient rapidly subside; mind clears, the headache becomes bearable, the eyes less sparkling, the swallowing less difficult, the intense redness of the skin fades. If all of these changes occur within a few hours after giving Belladonna to a case of scarlet fever that had been steadily growing worse up to the time that the drug was given, the most incredulous must admit that it is reasonable to believe that the subsidence of the symptoms must in some way be a sequence to the giving of the Belladonna. The fact that the one is the result of the other has been demonstrated millions of times by thousands of observers. By repeated experiments Hahnemann found that the theory held good when put to the practical test with a large number of drugs. Hence the law of cure was verified and shown to be as universal as the law of gravitation.

After the law of homeopathy was verified it was soon discovered that when drugs are given according to the homeopathic idea, it was not necessary to give them in large doses. Small doses were found to act more satisfactory. This peculiarity may be explained by the well-known fact that when our eyes are in a healthy condition the light of the brightest day does not affect them painfully, but if our eyes are inflamed we will be painfully conscious of the action of a single ray of light upon them. We reason by analogy, that when we are sick the smallest fraction of the drug whose physiological action is similar to the symptoms we possess, will be sufficient to affect us· But if we are well a much larger quantity is necessary to make an impression upon us. This explains the fact frequently cited by the opponents of homeopathy that they can eat an entire bottleful of homeopathic medicine and suffer no ill effect. Their statement will hold true in quite a number of properly prepared homeopathic remedies. But the fact has no weight whatever in proving that homeopathic remedies have no curative effect when administered to the sick. Homeopathic remedies are intended to cure the sick, not to make the well sick. The idea that a medicine, to be effective, must be highly colored, strong and nasty tasting, is an inheritance from barbarism. Belladonna is prepared for homeopathic use as follows: The *Deadly Nightshade*, a plant common in Europe, is gathered when coming into flower and the entire fresh plant is chopped and pounded to a fine pulp, enclosed in a piece of new linen and submitted to pressure. The expressed juice is then by brisk agitation mingled with an equal part by weight of alcohol. This mixture is allowed to stand eight days in a well stoppered bottle in a dark, cool place and then filtered, thus making the tincture which is a fluid resembling ordinary black coffee in color and consistency. Its drug power is said to be one-half, because it is one-half alcohol. Hence, two drops represent only one drop of the real tincture. Two parts are mixed with eight parts of alcohol and the resulting mixture is designated 1x or the first decimal dilution. One part of the first decimal dilution is mixed with nine parts of alcohol to make the 2x dilution. One part of the 2x dilution is mixed with nine parts of alcohol to make the 3x dilution, the potency or strength commonly used by homeopathic physicians. Some physicians claim they get good results even when they continue the process of diluting up to 30x or 200x. One drop of the 3x of Belladonna represents one thousandth of a drop of the tincture. Twenty drops of the 3x are usually put into half a glass of water, that is about twenty teaspoonsful. A teaspoonful is given at intervals ranging from ten minutes to two hours, according to the urgency of the case. In case of a convulsion the dose may be repeated every three minutes until relief. In very acute cases we have seen improvement follow in less than one minute after the administration of Belladonna. We have seen the scarlet face blanch within a few seconds. Old school physicians give Belladonna in doses ranging from ten to twenty drops of the tincture, repeated about every four hours. Thus it is readily figured out that their doses of Belladonna are *ten thousand* times as large as those of the homeopaths. All drugs, generally speaking, are poisons. To put into the system ten thousand times more of a drug than is actually necessary to bring about the desired result does not seem to us to be good practice. About the same difference exists between the old and the new school in reference to the doses of other drugs.

A few of the symptoms upon which both schools prescribe Belladonna are identical, but as a rule one school prescribes drugs never thought to be used in a given case by the other. Each year, however, sees the old school laying greater stress upon the physiological action of drugs and making their prescriptions accordingly. This seems to us to be the conclusion that all physicians must ultimately reach.

Belladonna pills or pellets are homeopathically prepared by saturating plain sugar of milk or cane sugar pills with a dilution of Belladonna, usually the 3x. The frequency of the repetition of the dose varies greatly with different remedies and in different cases, ranging from ten minutes to a week, but generally from every two to four hours.

Without going into the details of pharmacy we may say that other drugs obtained from plants are prepared in the same way as Belladonna. Drugs in powder form are prepared by using sugar of milk as the vehicle instead of alcohol. Both are neutral substances from a strictly medicinal point of view. The rubbing or grinding of a drug with sugar of milk is termed *triturating*. Hence we often speak of drugs after undergoing such a process as being of the 1x, 2x or 3x *trituration*, just as we speak of the 1x, 2x or 3x dilution when a drug has been diluted with alcohol. Homeopathic remedies are derived from the mineral, the vegetable and the animal kingdoms Bee poison, snake poisons, secretions from the deer (musk), and many other animal substances have been converted into valuable homeopathic remedies.

The homeopaths have made so many experiments or provings of so many drugs that it is scarcely possible now for one to have a sensation or a condition in any part of the body from the slightest to the gravest deviation from perfect health but that some remedy may be found in the homeopathic materia medica which has been observed to have produced upon a healthy person symptoms similar to yours. This is the reason that homeopaths rarely find it necessary to give opiates.

The homeopathic physician who knows his materia medica thoroughly is never at a loss for a remedy adapted to any symptoms he may meet. He may prescribe successfully for conditions and diseases he has not previously met. Before ever seeing a case of cholera, Hahnemann determined in advance what remedies would be most successful in combating the disease. He ascertained all the symptoms of cholera in its various stages, and knowing his materia medica, it was an easy matter for him to select Camphor, Cuprum, Veratrum Alb and Arsenicum. His prediction proved true, not only in the epidemic of his day, but in every succeeding epidemic; so true that statistics covering thousands and thousands of cases and including all the epidemics during the past one hundred years show that the death rate in cholera under homeopathic treatment has never reached ten per cent., while the rate among those under the old school treatment has rarely fallen below fifty per cent.

Homeopathic physicians distinguish, just as all other physicians should, the difference between medical and non-medical cases, that is, cases needing chiefly surgical, mechanical or hygienic treatment, and they act accordingly. It is a fact, however, that should be noted, that the patrons of homeopathy are less frequently compelled to undergo surgical operations than those who employ old school treatment.

Such a radical change in the practice of medicine as that introduced by Hahnemann naturally met with the most violent opposition in an age which was not characterized by such liberality as our own. Its author was ridiculed, ostracised and made to suffer beyond expression for his medical belief and practice. All schools now freely admit that if homeopathy has done nothing more, it has conferred an incalculable blessing upon humanity by compelling the old school to give smaller doses. It is believed that a century ago about as many were killed by huge doses of drugs as by disease. The friends of homeopathy know that it has accomplished more than the reduction of the size of the dose. At the recent congress of homeopathic physicians held in Chicago under the auspices of the auxilliary to the Columbian Exposition, statistics presented from twenty of the principal cities, representing one-fifteenth of the population of the United States, showed that the death rate among persons under homeopathic treatment was about *forty* per cent. less than it was among those who employed old school treatment. At this rate, if all sickness in the United States were treated homeopathically, the total number of deaths each year would be diminished nearly half a million. If each life be valued at $5,000 the difference between the two methods of treatment would amount to two and one-half billions. And this does not include the money paid out for drugs in quantities ten thousand times greater than is necessary.

While deserving the highest praise for its brilliant achievements in the the department of chemistry, bacteriology, pathology, surgery and preventive medicine, the old school must be severely criticised for its persistent neglect to utilize the superior therapeutic resources of homeopathy. If the old school physician constantly loses eight out of every one hundred of his scarlet fever patients, while the homeopathic physician as invariably loses but five, is not the former rightly blamed for the loss of three lives if he does not utilize the treatment of his homeopathic neighbor? In fact, ought not the law to compel him to give his patients the treatment that has been repeatedly demonstrated to possess such superiority?

Reader, we know you would think so if one of those three unnecessarily fatal cases were a child of yours. We would suggest to our conscientious allopathic brother that he consider his responsbility under such circumstances.

Chemistry, microscopy and bacteriology have recently revealed the fact that the germs of the most deadly diseases are so small as to be lost within a blood corpuscle three thousandth of an inch in diameter. The day of ridiculing or underestimating the power of small things is past. The homeopathic physicians of today have little opposition compared with those of the earlier followers of Hahnemann. They are 15,000 strong in the United States. They number some twenty colleges and thirty journals. They have control of about a hundred hospitals, asylums, sanitariums and dispensaries. They have representation on nearly every State board of health in the Union. Their peculiar belief is taught at the expense of the State in three State universities, namely: Michigan, Iowa and Minnesota, and their patrons are numbered by increasing millions.

The clientage of the homeopathic physician, other things being equal, is invariably better than that of his allopathic brother practicing in the same locality. When he retires at night the homeopathic physician has the comforting assurance that he has not given any poor sufferer an overdose of some poisonous drug, but to all who have been so wise as to place their health and their lives in his keeping he has given that medicine which will cure in the easiest manner and the speediest time possible.

Supposed Incurables.

There are thousands of persons supposed to be incurable who are capable of being entirely and permanently cured. The boundary line between the curable and the incurable is not and never will be fixed or well defined.

The following cases are reported here, not for the purpose of vaunting the skill of the authors, nor for the purpose of exposing the ignorance of others; not to inspire with false hope the few that are really incurable, but to encourage the many who are absolutely curable, but who, laboring under the impression that they have faithfully tried everything in vain, are resigned to suffer unnecessarily the remainder of their existence.

To all such we would say, no matter how many physicians you have consulted, no matter how many kinds of treatment you have tried, no matter how much medicine you have taken, the probabilities are ten to one that you have made less than half an effort to get well.

A reputable physician recently told us that he had just cured a case of insanity of thirteen years' standing and that he was the seventy-ninth physician that had been consulted. The cure was effected by a surgical operation.

We never saw the patient and cannot vouch for the doctor's statements, but we did see and read the letter which remitted with thanks his fee of two thousand dollars.

We can, however, vouch for the following reports, because the cases were under our personal care:

Case I.—Clara S., aged 20, a farmer's daughter. Health always good until she slid down from a load of hay. She was brought to Chicago October 1, 1892. She had then been confined to bed eleven months. She did not bring her shoes along because it was not expected that she would ever walk again. After three months of local treatment, massage, electricity and the indicated homeopathic remedies, she began to walk. Six months later she could outwalk all her friends who came to visit the World's Fair with her. In a recent letter she states that she is entirely well and is happily married.

Case II.—Mrs. Paul M., age 35, was confined to her bed the greater part of the time from October 1892 to April 1893 with what was called womb trouble, the pain being so intense that much of the time she was kept under the influence of morphine. Thirty treatments with galvanism, along with the indicated homeopathic remedies, extending over a period of two months, cured her so that she could resume her duties as a teacher.

Case III.—Miss P. C., possessing an unusually good intellect, graduated at Oxford college in 1877. During the next six years she was a teacher in that institution. Easter Sunday, 1883, she fainted in church, and during the next ten years she was confined to her bed the greater part of the time with what was called spinal trouble. For seven years previous to May 1, 1893, she rarely sat up and when she did, it was usually for a period of not longer than fifteen minutes.

For seven years her meals were carried to her. For seven years she did not touch her piano of which she was very fond. For seven years she did not walk up or down stairs. For seven years she had not been out of doors, except when carried out. Her spine was exceedingly sensitive from one extremity to the other. It took her fifteen minutes to turn herself over in bed and the effort caused her intense agony.

Physician after physician saw her. Every one gave a guarded or discouraging prognosis. A physician, a college president who has a national reputation, after making his fourth examination, said to her: "My dear woman, you have called me to tell you the truth, and it pains me exceedingly to be obliged to say to you that there is not a physician on earth skillful enough to enable you to walk again." She and her friends were given to understand, not only by this physician but by another nearly as eminent, that she must content herself to being confined to her bed the remainder of her days.

When, the first of last June, we told the patient that she would visit the World's Fair our integrity was questioned by her family, because they considered our statement the most extravagant and irrational that they had ever known a medical man to make. She visited the Fair three times. The first time, August 27th. The second time, September 22nd, on which day she walked five hours, visiting every room on the first floor of the Art Building. She now attends receptions, weddings, entertainments, and often goes to church twice on Sunday. During the past winter she has walked out daily, rain or shine. Surgery, massage, electricity, dietetics and homeopathy have accomplished her recovery.

The essential facts in this remarkable and almost incredible case could be substantiated by hundreds of persons, and by no less a personage than the distinguished preacher, Prof. David Swing, of Chicago, who has known the patient from childhood.

Case IV.—Bessie L., now age 14, was a healthy, bright, active, school girl until November 1892, when she was taken out of school on account of failing health. She complained of being tired, of backache, and sat around in a listless manner. She gradually grew worse, and by May 1, 1893, she was confined to her bed, unable to walk or even to raise her head. Her spine was now extremely sensitive throughout its entire length. During the summer and autumn she had frequent convulsions in which her head and feet bent backwards until they nearly met. She would remain drawn in this agonizing position for hours at a time. For two months last fall her hands were fixed behind her while her legs were drawn up under her in an immovable position. About the first of December Prof. L. H. Anderson hypnotized her. Her arms and legs were straightened out, and in the course of a few weeks she regained considerable use of the hands. During December and January she was hypnotized about twice a week. It required but a few seconds to put her into the hypnotic state. On several occasions when she was hypnotized her body was so rigid that she could be lifted up horizontally, supported only at the head and feet. While hypnotism benefited her more than anything previously tried, it failed to cure. To detail all the efforts made by the distressed parents of this afflicted girl to have her cured would fill a volume. Fifteen physicians were consulted. A stay in one of the large hospitals resulted in nothing more than her being filled with morphine. From May to December fifty-seven Spanish fly blisters were applied to her spine. These were soothing compared with the constant, terrible pain in her back and she often cried to have them put on.

On the 24th of February she was brought into our private home as helpless as an infant. She could not walk nor turn over. She could not even move her head. The muscles of the neck which control the movements of the head were absolutely powerless. She would lie exactly in whatever position placed until moved. Her spine was so sensitive that the slightest touch at any point would cause her to cry out. This was true even when she was asleep and also when she was in the hypnotic state.

On the 4th of March, in the presence of six physicians[†] who had previously examined her, we operated, with ether as an anæsthetic. An attempt to use hypnotism instead failed, because the patient suspected what we were about to do and rebelled. She said that she would not be hypnotized and she was not, though Prof. Anderson tried for an hour.

Notwithstanding the fact that the operation was very severe the evidences of improvement were soon apparent. During the entire period of her sickness she was never known to sleep in the day time, and it often required a hypnotic to make her sleep at night, but during the first week after the operation she slept, on the average, eighteen hours out of every twenty-four. The urine, instead of being scanty or suppressed as formerly, became profuse. The hands and feet became warm and pinkish instead of cold and clammy as before the operation. On the 17th day of March she raised her head and stood alone. On the 20th, while the nurse was out, she dressed herself and walked down two flights of stairs, something she had not done for sixteen months, and today, the 24th of March, twenty days

---

[†]Among those present were Dr. W. H. Burt, Dr. Julia Holmes Smith, and Dr. Richard Dewey, ex-superintendent of Kankakee Insane Asylum.

after the operation, she has walked a quarter of a mile on the streets. Now, instead of moaning and crying, as formerly, during the greater part of her waking hours, she laughs, sings and even attempts to dance. Not a trace of the tenderness of the spine remains and permanent restoration of health may now be predicted with a positive certainty.

INDEX OF SUBJECTS.

A.

Abortion, 299.
Abscess, 283.
Acne, 257
Actinomycosis, 113.
Addison's Disease, 180.
Adenitis, 98.
Albuminuria, 187.
Albuminoids, 304.
Alcoholism, 236.
Amenorrhœa, 208.
Anæsthetics, 284.
Anæmia, 180, 227.
Aneurism, 179.
Angina Pectoris, 178.
Anthrax, 80.
Antiseptic Precaution, 284.
Aphasia, 229.
Apoplexy, 227.
Appendicitis, 151.
Arsenical Poisoning, 238.
Arthritis Deformans, 123.
Arteries, 179.
Ascaris Lumbricoides, 242.
Ascites, 157.
Asparagus, 315.
Asthma, 165.
Asiatic Cholera, 69.
Atony of Bladder, 197.

B.

Baby, 300.
Baked Beans, 314.
Basedow's Disease, 183.
Bed Sore, 288.
Bi-Chloride, 281.
Bladder, 196.
Black-Heads, 262.
Blepharitis, 266.
Blood, 78, 180, 183.
Blues, 250.
Boils, 288.
Bones, Broken, 292.
Boric Acid, 282.
Brain, 223.
Breasts, 297.
Bowels, 146.
Bright's Disease, 190.
Bronchitis, 163.
Bronchi, 163.
Bronchiectasis, 165.
Bubo, 87.
Burns, 260, 291.

C.

Cancer, 145.
Carbolic Acid, 282.
Carbuncle, 289.
Catarrh, 159.
Cataract, 272.
Cerebro Spinal Fever, 49.
Cereals, 314.
Characteristics, 321.
Child Bed Fever, 78, 296.
Chicken Pox, 13.
Cholera, 69.
Cholera Infantum, 147.
Chlorosis, 180.
Chorea, 230.
Choroid, 273.
Chloroform, 286.
Circumcision, 301.
Cirrhosis, 155.
Clap, 201.

Comedo, 262.
Continued Remittent Fever, 55.
Consumption, 99.
Constipation, 153.
Congestion of Lungs, 166.
Conception, 207, 293.
Convulsions, 230, 301.
Conjunctiva, 267.
Contusions, 290.
Confinement. 295.
Cord, 300.
Croup, 162.
Crystaline Lens, 272.

D.

Decomposition, 281.
Desquamation, 16.
Dengue Fever, 60.
Delusions, 244.
Dermatitis, 259.
Diphtheria, 24.
Dilutions, 7.
Diabetes, 123, 125.
Dietetics, 303.
Dilatation of Stomach, 144.
Dilutions, 319.
Diuretin, 158.
Displacement of Womb, 210.
Dose, 318.
Dropsy, 157.
Dysentery, 107.
Dysmenorrhœa, 209.

E.

Ear, 275.
Eczema, 253.
Ectropion, 266.
Embolism, 228.
Emphysema, 173.
Endo-carditis, 176.
Endo-metritis, 212.
Encephalitis, 229.
Enteritis, 147.
Entropion, 266.
Ephermeral Fever, 113.
Epilepsy, 231.
Epistaxis, 160.
Erosion, 215.
Eruptive Fevers, 12.
Erysipelas, 76.

Ether, 286.
Eucalyptus, 282.
Evidences of Health, 3.
Exophthalmic Goitre, 183.
Eye, 266.

F.

Fats, 304, 313.
Fatty Degeneration, 178.
Febricula, 113.
Felon, 284, 289.
Fevers, 11.
Fever Diet, 312.
Fibroid, 216.
Fibroid Phthisis, 102.
Flexions of Womb, 211.
Flesh Diet, 311.
Flesh Worms, 262.
Fractures, 292.
Fruits, 316.

G.

Gangrene, 171, 280, 289.
Gastritis, 139.
Gastralgia, 143.
Gastrodinia, 145.
Gaul Stone, 154.
German Measles, 110.
Glanders, 112.
Glaucoma, 274.
Goitre, 183.
Gout, 121.
Gonococcus, 201.
Gonorrhœa, 201.
Gonorrhœal Rheumatism, 117.
Grain Poisoning, 240.
Grand Mal, 231.
Graves' Disease, 183.

H.

Hahnemann, 5.
Hæmatemesis, 145.
Hæmaturia, 186.
Hallucination, 244.
Hæmorrhage, 40, 290.
Hæmorrhage of Stomach, 145.
Hæmorrhage of Lungs, 167.
Hæmorrhage of Bladder, 186.
Hæmorrhage of Kidneys, 186.
Hæmorrhage of Child Birth, 298.

Hæmophilia, 129.
Hæmoptysis, 167.
Heart, 176.
Headache, 223.
Hematocele, 217.
Hemiplegia, 228.
Hernia, 291.
Herpes, 262.
Hives, 261.
Hodgkin's Disease, 182.
Hydrophobia, 81.
Hydropericardium, 176.
Hypertrophy of Heart, 177.
Hyperæmia of Brain, 227.
Hydro-nephrosis, 195.
Hydro-thorax, 172.
Hysteria, 233.

I.

Illusions, 244.
Imperative Conceptions, 245.
Indicanuria, 189.
Inflammation, 281.
Influenza, 62.
Insanity, 244.
Injuries and Repair, 280.
Inspissated Cerumen, 275.
Intermittent Fever, 53.
Intestinal Obstruction, 152.
Iodoform, 282.
Iritis, 271.
Iridectomy, 274.
Irritation, 281.
Itch, 260.

J.

Jacksonian Epilepsy, 232.
Jaundice, 154.
Joints, 292.

K.

Keratitis, 271.
Kidneys, 185.
Kumyss, 310.

L.

La Grippe, 62.
Laceration, 215.
Larynx, 161.
Laryngitis, 161.

Leprosy, 111.
Lead Poisoning, 237.
Leukæmia, 181.
Leucorrhœa, 213.
Lids, 266.
Lithæmia, 122, 188.
Liver, 154.
Lock Jaw, 85.
Local Tuberculosis, 98.
Locomotor Ataxia, 222.
Localization, 229.
Lumbago, 118.
Lungs, 166.
Lumpy Jaw, 113.

M.

Malarial Fever, 53.
Malta Fever, 115.
Matzoon, 310.
Materia Medica, 318.
Measles, 18.
Meat, 310.
Mediastinum, 174.
Melancholia, 247.
Meningitis, 49, 226.
Meningeal Tuberculosis, 97.
Menstruation, 208.
Menorrhagia, 209.
Metritis, 215.
Metrorrhagia, 209.
Milk Sickness, 114.
Milk, 309.
Mind, 244.
Miscarriage, 299.
Mountain Fever, 115.
Mother and Child, 293.
Morning Sickness, 293.
Monomania, 248.
Morphia Habit, 237.
Mumps, 65.
Muscular Rheumatism, 118.
Myalgia, 117.
Myocarditis, 177.
Myxœdema, 183.

N.

Nervous System, 220.
Nervous Dyspepsia, 143.
Nephritis, 190.
Nephrolithiasis, 195.

Nettle Rash, 261.
Neuralgia, 232.
Neurasthenia, 235.
Neuritis, 220.
Neurosis, 143.
Neuromata, 221.
Nose, 160.

O.

Oatmeal, 314.
Obesity, 242.
Obstruction of Bowels, 152.
Œsophagus, 138.
Olfactory Nerve, 221.
Ophthalmia, 268.
Opiates, 9.
Optic Nerve, 221.
Otorrhœa, 278.
Ovaralgia, 218.
Ovaritis, 218.
Ovarian Tumor, 219.
Oxaluria, 189.

P.

Paliatives, 9.
Palpitation, 178.
Pancreas, 156.
Paralysis Agitans, 230.
Paretic Dementia, 247.
Patent Medicine, 8.
Pernicious Malarial Fever, 56.
Peptic Ulcer, 144.
Peritoneum, 156.
Peritonitis, 157.
Pericardium, 175.
Pericarditis, 175.
Perinephric Abscess, 196.
Pellets, 318-319.
Pelvic Cellulitis, 216.
Pelvic Peritonitis. 216.
Pelvic Abscess, 217.
Pelvic Hematocele, 217.
Petit Mal, 231.
Periodical Insanity, 248.
Pediculosis, 258.
Peroxide, 283.
Perineum, 298.
Pharmacy, 318-320.
Phosphaturia, 189.
Phthisis, 99.

Pleura, 172.
Pleurisy, 172.
Pneumonia, 168.
Pneumonothorax, 173.
Pneumonokoniosis, 172.
Poisonings, 236.
Polypus, 338.
Potencies, 319-321.
Premature Labor, 299.
Pregnancy, 293.
Prevention of Conception, 207.
Prevention of disease, 9.
Professional Spasms, 233.
Pruritus, 261.
Psoriasis, 258.
Ptomaine, 239.
Pterygium, 270.
Ptyalism, 133.
Pulmonary Tuberculosis. 97.
Pulmonary Hemorrhage, 167.
Pulse, 4.
Purpura, 128.
Purpura Hemorrhagica, 129.
Pyelitis, 194.
Pyæmia, 79.
Pyuria, 187.

R.

Relapsing Fever, 52.
Renal Sclerosis, 191.
Respiratory System, 159.
Retina, 273.
Retention of Urine, 296.
Rheumatism. 116.
Rheumatic Neuralgia, 119.
Rickets, 126.
Ring Worm, 259.
Rules of Diet, 316.
Rupture, 291.

S.

Saint Vitus Dance, 230.
Salpingitis, 217.
Salisbury's Experiments, 314.
Scalds, 291.
Scabies, 260.
Scarlet Fever, 14.
Sciatica, 221.
Scorbutus, 127.
Scurvy, 127.

Scrofula, 98.
Septicæmia, 78.
Self Abuse, 204.
Sexual Abuse, 204.
Senile Dementia, 247.
Seborrhœa, 263.
Senile Gangrene, 280, 289.
Shaking Palsy, 230.
Shock, 289.
Sick Headache, 223.
Skin, 251.
Small-pox, 21.
Spermatorrhœa, 206.
Spinal Cord, 222.
Spectacles, 272.
Splints, 292.
Sprains 291.
Statistics, 6.
Starches, 313.
Starch, 304.
Stomach, 139.
Stomatitis, 131.
Stone in Bladder, 200.
Suralimentation, 103.
Sub-Acute Rheumatism, 118.
Suicidal Poisoning, 240.
Sun Stroke, 241.
Surgery, Principles of, 279.
Suppuration, 283.
Syphilis, 84.
Syphilitic Rheumatism, 118.
Sweating Sickness, 115.

T.

Table of Foods, 307.
Tænia Saginata, 243.
Tape Worm, 243.
Temperature, 4.
Tetanus, 85.
Tetany, 233.
Tetter, 253.
Thrombosis, 228.
Tinea Trichophytina, 259.
Throat, 134.

Thyroid Gland, 183.
Tonsillitis, 135.
Traumatic Neurosis, 235.
Trichiniasis, 242.
Triturations, 319-321.
Tumors, 216.
Tumors of Brain, 229.
Tuberculosis, 93.
Typhoid fever, 34, 44.

U.

Ulcers, 288.
Unclassified Affections, 236.
Uræmia, 189.
Urine, Normal, 3.
Urine, Retention, 197.
Urine, Suppression, 197.
Urine, Incontinence, 198.
Urinary Fistula, 203.
Urethra, 196.
Urethritis, 197.
Urticaria, 261.

V.

Valvular Diseases, 177.
Version of Womb, 211.
Vesical Tenesmus, 198.
Vegetarians, 311.
Vicarious Menstruation, 209.
Vitreous Humor, 274.

W.

Water, 308.
Ways of Cure, 5.
What is Disease? 4.
White Blood Corpuscles, 28
Whooping Cough, 66.
Women, Diseases of, 208.
Wounds, 281.
Wry-neck, 118.

Y.

Yellow Fever, 46.

Up to Date!

CONTAINS ALL THE N. IDEAS IN MEDICINE A1 SURGERY. . . . . .

Describes all Diseases.   Explains their Causes.

THIS IS THE **LATEST** Family Medical Book.

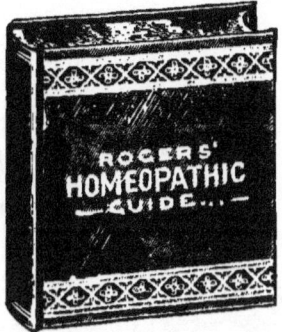

Gives numerous invaluable suggestions for their prevention, along with the best method of treatment. Discusses more fully than any other similar work, the subject of Dietetics, Insanity, Nervous Diseases, Skin Diseases, the Baby, Diseases of Women and Children, the Relation of the Sexes and the Diseases peculiar to them. Written by Drs. L. D. and Ida Wright Rogers, in plain language which any one can understand. Contains 370 pages, handsomely bound and clearly printed on extra good paper. Price, only *One Dollar* including a year's subscription to the PEOPLE'S HEALTH JOURNAL

READ WHAT THEY HAVE TO SAY:

John Bower, Sylvester, Mich.: I like Rogers' Guide very much.

Mrs. Bell Shoemaker, Melford, Ia.: The more I read it the better I like it.

Dr. E. S. Evans, Columbus, O.: It is good. The arrangement is par excellence.

J. M Reid, Chatham, Ont.: It is concise, thorough, and worded in a readable manner.

A. J. Sweet, Clifton, Kan.: I would not take $10 for my new medical book if I could not get another.

Cyrus D. Henry, Canandaigua, N. Y.: Rogers' Homeopathic Guide more perfectly meets our needs than anything I had dared hope to find. My trouble as a layman has been to decide on the proper medicine. The Guide's materia medica is the most tangible of anything I ever saw.

Rev. H. O. Rowlands, D. D., Chicago: Brief and lucid. No verbosity. Every statement to the point. Everything conveyed in plain words with the elegance of simplicity and directness, so that the mother and nurse will have no difficulty in understanding the symptoms and treatment of diseases.

The Homeopathic Physician, Philadelphia: A veritable miniature encyclopedia of diseases and their treatment. It might be studied with profit by practitioners, especially beginners and students.

Dr. J. H. S. Johnson, Chicago: It actually contains more than works twice the size, and gives the diagnosis and treatment of many diseases which no other domestic work mentions. I have never read a volume wherein so much is told in so few words.

Address the **PEOPLE'S HEALTH JOURNAL**, CHICAGO.

TRAINED NURSE.

Young women possessing intelligence, strength and good health, cannot enter a better field than that of a trained nurse. It is about the only one that is not overcrowded. The occupation is one peculiarly suited for women. The demand for trained female nurses is greater than the supply. The wages range from $15 to $25 a week. No young woman will make a mistake in acquiring a thorough knowledge of nursing. Such knowledge will some day serve her to the greatest advantage. The opportunity will come when knowledge of this character will outweigh any other accomplishment she may possess. We have a plan by which you can become an accomplished and practical nurse without leaving your home. Let every young woman who has any spare time, write us for information, "How to Become a Trained Nurse at Home." Address with two cent stamp:

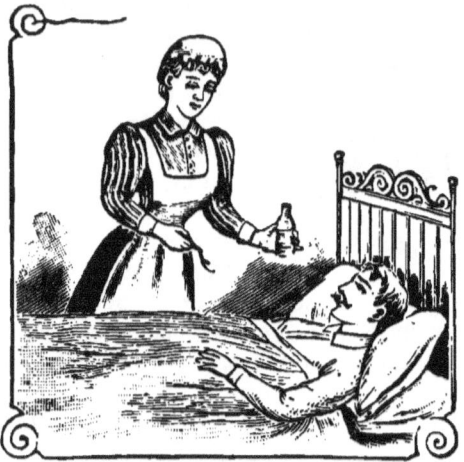

PEOPLE'S HEALTH JOURNAL CO., Chicago, Ill.

You Can Study Medicine At Home.

You can study medicine at home advantageously. You can also save a year's time. Write us for full particulars, "How to Begin the Study of Medicine."

ADDRESS:

PEOPLE'S HEALTH JOURNAL,

CHICAGO.

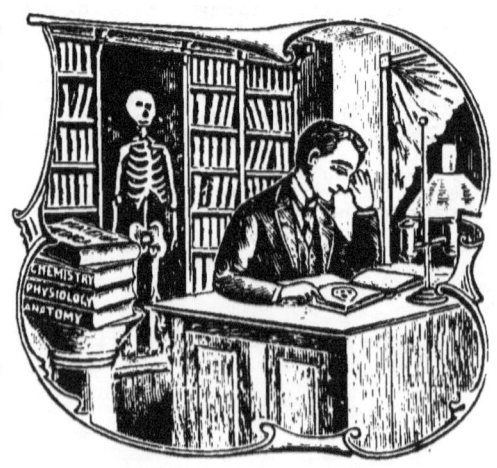

Homeopathic Family Medicine Chest Free.

A FAMILY MEDICINE CHEST, strongly made, of Spanish cedar, having nails, hinges and fastenings of brass, and containing 24 two drachm bottles, labeled and filled with the most commonly used remedies, accompanied with plain directions, when and how to use them, will be sent to any address, expressage or delivery charges prepaid, and the PEOPLE'S HEALTH JOURNAL regularly for one year for only *One Dollar*.

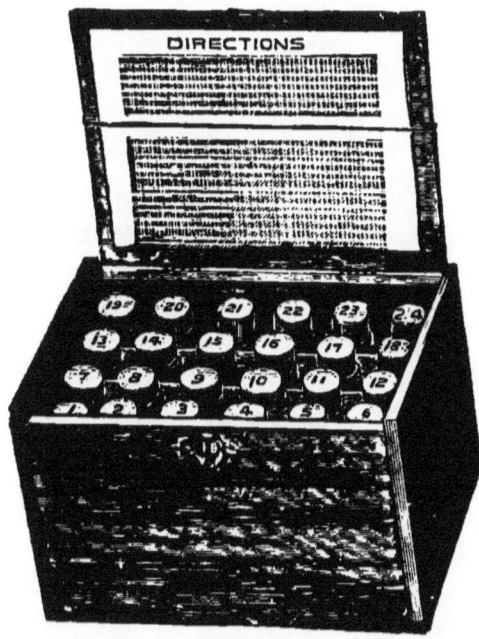

We believe this offer has never been equalled. The price of a single bottle of medicine, the size of one of these 24, would be, at almost any retail drug store, 25 cents. At which rate 24 would cost $6.00, to say nothing of the chest, the directions, and the convenience of having such a supply of medicines at hand ready for any emergency such as croup, convulsions, colic, chill, or the first stage of a "cold" when relief must be had at once, when it may be inconvenient or undesirable to call a physician, and at a time when "a stitch in time saves nine." Many a family have saved money, time, worry, suffering, and even life by having such a chest at hand. Should be in every home. 17,000 families have one. Mothers prize it.

Frank T. R. Long, of Elizaville, Ind., in the following letter, dated March 24, 1894, expresses what thousands have written us during the past few years: "I take pleasure in acknowledging the receipt of the Medicine Chest that you give as a premium with the JOURNAL. The chest and medicines go far beyond my expectations. I consider that you give four times the value of the subscription price of your paper ($1 00). As I am a salesman for all kinds of homeopathic remedies, I know that the cost of this chest is far more than you charge for both. It is a wonder how you can offer this expensive outfit for less than $3.00.

Address: **PEOPLE'S HEALTH JOURNAL,** Chicago.

www.ingramcontent.com/pod-product-compliance
Lightning Source LLC
Chambersburg PA
CBHW020311240426
43673CB00039B/767